GERIATRIC
PSYCHIATRY
BASICS

A NORTON PROFESSIONAL BOOK

GERIATRIC PSYCHIATRY BASICS

Kenneth Sakauye, MD

W. W. Norton & Company
New York · London

For information about permission to reproduce selections from this book,
write to Permissions, W. W. Norton & Company, Inc., 500 Fifth Avenue, New York,
NY 10110

For information about special discounts for bulk purchases, please contact
W. W. Norton Special Sales at specialsales@wwnorton.com or 800-233-4830.

Composition by Anna Oler
Manufacturing by Malloy
Production Manger: Leeann Graham

Library of Congress Cataloging-in-Publication Data

Sakauye, Kenneth M.
Geriatric psychiatry basics: a handbook for general psychiatrists /
Kenneth Sakauye. — 1st ed.
p. ; cm.
"A Norton Professional Book."
Includes bibliographical references and index.
ISBN 978-0-393-70501-0 (pbk.)
1. Geriatric psychiatry—Handbooks, manuals, etc. I. Title. [DNLM: 1. Aged. 2.
Mental Disorders—therapy. 3. Geriatric Psychiatry—methods. WT 150 S158g 2008]
RC451.4.A5S23 2008
618.97'689—dc22   2007021086

W. W. Norton & Company, Inc.
500 Fifth Avenue, New York, N.Y. 10110
www.wwnorton.com

W. W. Norton & Company Ltd.
Castle House, 75/76 Wells St., London W1T 3QT

1 3 5 7 9 8 6 4 2 0

*To the survivors of Katrina,
who so strongly influenced
my life and thinking.*

CONTENTS

ACKNOWLEDGMENTS

Although a bevy of individuals helped in the writing of this book, my fondest indebtedness goes to the mentors in my professional life.

First, I want to thank Shilpa Srinivasan, M.D., now on faculty at the University of South Carolina, whose fellowship was interrupted by Hurricane Katrina and who reviewed initial drafts of chapters as part of her "training;" my wife Beverly, who kindly read all chapters from a lay person's perspective to be sure sections were readable; and Andrea Costella, my editor, who gently shaped the format and revisions.

My ideas were influenced most by Robert L. Kahn, Ph.D. at the University of Chicago, who introduced me to geriatrics and was like a second father to me; George Pollock, M.D., the former Head of the Chicago Psychoanalytic Institute, who helped shape much of my thinking about psychotherapy with the elderly; and Mary Harper, RN, Ph.D., who was one of the first black women to serve at an executive level at the National Institute of Mental Health (NIMH), and who taught me by involving me in committees and being a mentor from a distance.

PREFACE

In my experience, many residents in general psychiatry training programs, psychiatrists, and mental health professionals who are not involved in geriatrics often start out with the stereotypes that dementia and depression are normal conditions of old age, rather than disease states, and therefore have an unjustified therapeutic nihilism. There is often confusion about what is normal and what is pathological. Early dementia is often overdiagnosed when changes are more likely to be due to an undiagnosed depression or medication side effect. Common psychosocial issues are not investigated. Often atypical presentations and overlapping findings from medical illness make psychiatric diagnosis difficult. A generation gap seems to exist between the older patient and the younger doctor.

This primer is meant to address the more commonly encountered issues in geriatric psychiatry for the general psychiatrist, and other clinicians and counselors who work with geriatric patients. It should also have importance for the general medical practitioner who is the first line of treatment for older adults.

Geriatric care is characterized by many unique factors: (1) It requires knowledge of neuroscience and neurological and medical information; (2) it must be multidisciplinary; (3) it involves more contact with families; and (4) it is the testing ground for new reimbursement policies by the largest insurer in the United States—Medicare. Norms and psychological issues seem to differ from those of younger adults and require at least passing knowledge of sociological and psychological information. Psychotherapy techniques often need to be modified to accommodate sensory impairment or mild cognitive impairment. Indeed, the frequency of cognitive impairment requires knowledge about the various dementias and delirium. Prescribing practices have unique rules, and issues of institutional care and changing family dynamics are also specific to this population.

This book has been delayed by a full year due to my personal experience of Hurricane Katrina, which wreaked havoc on the health-care infrastructure and universities in New Orleans and caused a hiatus in my professional life. I was a professor of clinical psychiatry at Louisiana State University (LSU) Medical School, clinical professor of psychiatry at Tulane Medical School, and director of geriatric psychiatry at LSU and Ochsner Foundation Hospital in New Orleans before August, 2005. I am now building geriatric services and a geriatric psychiatry fellowship at the University of Tennessee Health Science Center, College of Medicine, where I am a professor of psychiatry and vice-chair of clinical affairs in Memphis. A part of me welcomed the move, but another part still misses New Orleans.

In the Katrina aftermath, in addition to dealing with personal and family needs, I spent a large amount of time trying to restore services in New Orleans and working with the elderly and their families who returned. The American Association for Geriatric Psychiatry (AAGP), where I served on the executive committee, responded to my appeal to provide funding support for a Disaster Task Force to develop guidelines for treating elderly disaster victims, to avoid repeating the neglect and errors in the care of frail elderly and dementia patients post-Katrina. In this primer I hesitated to write a chapter on Katrina, because the problem and interventions are beyond even social psychiatry. It is not about service delivery per se, but a societal challenge. The majority of deaths from Katrina occurred in elderly populations, especially minority elderly. Post-Katrina frail elderly regressed, and reports of suicides and excess mortality increased. Issues of abandonment, separation from the familiar, and limited resources to provide comfort and safety took center stage in New Orleans, but these very challenges highlighted for all mental health professionals across the country how we can better care for our elderly. Although not always viewed as a psychiatric intervention, instilling hope and helping plan for the future are major interventions.

Disaster can also be a learning experience. I hope, with this book, I have been able to incorporate a common-sense and empathic approach to evidence-based care for the elderly—an approach that I believe was shaped in large part based on my experiences with Katrina.

GERIATRIC
PSYCHIATRY
BASICS

1

SUCCESSFUL AGING AND APPLICATION OF THE BIOPSYCHOSOCIAL MODEL

The field of geriatric psychiatry comprises the special body of knowledge about older adults that is usually not covered well in residents' general adult training. This knowledge includes:

- Late-life development
- Biology of aging
- Common medical illnesses associated with aging
- Neurobiology of degenerative disorders
- Geriatric psychopharmacology
- Psychotherapeutic modifications for special populations, such as patients with cognitive impairment
- Heightened skill in coordinating multidisciplinary care and family involvement
- Knowledge of health-care policies (e.g., knowledge of Medicare, guidelines such as Healthy People 2010, retirement issues)
- Familiarity with housing options, supportive services, and nursing home reform
- Specific studies of older adults as a special population (differences)
- Public health issues concerning health-care disparities of older adults, perhaps especially patients from minority groups

There is a demographic imperative to deal with our older adult population. That is, the growing numbers of older adults, especially those living to advanced age, have resulted in a situation in which most general psychiatrists provide care for older adults in their practice, and are usually the first to receive a geriatric patient referral from primary care physicians. Likewise, primary care physicians are expected to recognize and treat geriatric psychiatry issues before they refer. This book cannot cover all of the geriatric issues of which a specialist must be aware, but instead offers a primer on the salient topics and geriatric disorders a practitioner is likely to face.

The demographics were already changing by 1950 due to reduced infant mortality and higher longevity. When graphed by age, the pattern looked like a pyramid with the largest age group being children and progressive population decline by age due to mortality (see Figure 1.1). With a projected decrease in birth rates and family size and continued improvements in mortality rates, the graph is beginning to look more like a rectangle with equal age distributions, not more children (see Figure 1.2). If the trend continues with low birth rates and increased longevity, the future may portend an aged society with few children and mainly older adults—an inverted pyramid. U.S. census data over the last 50 years show the changing graph.

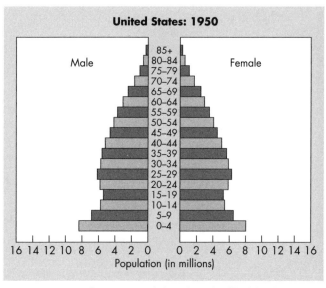

Figure 1.1. Classic, pyramid-shaped graph of high birth rate
and high mortality.
Source: From U.S. Census Bureau (2000).

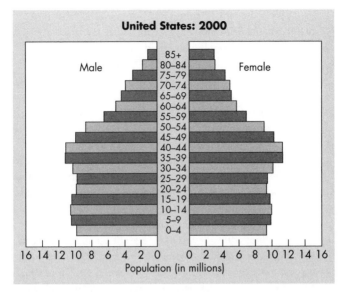

Figure 1.2. Inverted pyramid shaped graph of low birth rate
and low death rate.
Source: From U.S. Census Bureau (2000).

Other demographic information on older adults from the
2000 U.S. Census reveals the following:

- Those 75 and over represented 35% of the older population;
  those 85 and over represented 12% of the older population
  and had the highest percentage increase among the older
  population, increasing by 38% to 4.2 million individuals.
- Women outnumbered men by growing margins from age 65;
  in the age group 65–74 there were 83 men to every 100
  women; in the age group 85 and over there were only 46
  men to every 100 women.
- More than half of the older population was married: 74% of
  men and 45% of women between ages 65 and 84 were married; 41% of women in this age group were widowed. Above
  age 85, 58% of men and 12% of women were married; 79%
  of women in this age group are widowed.
- 71% of those ages 65–84 had completed high school; 58% of

those 85 and over had completed 9th grade; 27% of those over 85 had a 9th-grade or less education.

- 20% of married-couple households with a householder 65 and older had an income below $20,000; 48.9% had incomes $35,000 or more (higher than the national average). (Social Security usually ensures that older adults live above the poverty line, but if this is the only source of income, it barely exceeds poverty level.)
- Of five disabilities measured by the census in 2000 (sensory, physical, mental, self-care, ambulation) there were at least three times the rate of the total population (physical, sensory, ambulation); 47% of the population over age 85 reported a disability that caused difficulties going outside the home, and 28% showed problems learning, remembering, or concentrating.
- 1.8% of older adults between the ages of 65 and 74 lived in group quarters (mainly nursing homes), and 21.9% of those 85 and older lived in group quarters. Overall, 5.7% of those 65+ lived in group quarters. Over age 85, 39.2% lived with others in a household, and 38.9% still lived alone.
- There are proportionately fewer older adults from minority groups than younger populations because of immigration patterns and early mortality. The percentage of non-Hispanic whites was 80% for ages 65–74, and 87% for those 85 and older.

The old saying that the true test of a society is how well it treats its prisoners and old people is highly applicable at this point in U.S. history.

"NORMAL" AGING

A central question about aging is which changes are normal and which are related to disease processes? For example, is the tendency of many older adults to reminisce and repeat themselves a normal process of a life review in consolidating their sense of self as roles and health change, or is it an early sign of dementia? Cultural differences of normal aging add to the complexity. For example, Hispanics from lower socioeconomic strata (SES; lower education and unskilled labor) often view the 50s as old, whereas middle-class Northern European Americans tend to view the 80s as old age. Many older patients say that they have "old-timers disease" for what they view as normal memory loss with age. Defining "normal aging" can be an ambiguous task.

The first rule in geriatric psychiatry is that just because something happens frequently does not make it normal. For example, Alzheimer's disease may occur in almost 50% of older adults by their mid-80s, but it is still not normal, and it is a potentially treatable disease. Similarly, behavior disturbances that occur with Alzheimer's disease (AD) are never "normal," even though behavioral problems occur in possibly 85% of AD patients. Living to 100 in good physical and mental health might be rare, but it is still "normal." Normal aging generally involves changes that occur universally, that are usually not noticeable to the individual, and that do not cause disability or impairment.

Longitudinal studies are better than cross-sectional studies in determining normative (common) changes in functions, from young adulthood to old age, on an individual basis. However, because such long-term studies are costly and so many problems exist in interpreting the findings, very few exist. Examples of external influences that can impede generalizations are the effect of history (e.g., wars); individual differences (e.g., life crises, personality); instruments used to measure change; culture; family structure; and statistical methods. Some of the main longitudinal studies that have provided the best information are the Harvard Study of Adult Development (Vaillant, 2003), the Berkeley Guidance Study and Oakland Growth (Carolina Population Center, 2006), the Yale study of men from young to middle adulthood (Levinson, Darrow, & Klein, 1978), the Duke OARS (Older Americans Resources and Services; 2006), and the Baltimore Longitudinal Study of Aging (National Institute of Health, 2007). Participants in cross-sectional studies may be contacted after many years have passed to obtain a new wave of data to create longitudinal information. A less useful method is to make inferences from longitudinal data collected over shorter time periods (i.e., repeating measurements sooner).

Changes that are common with advancing age are listed in Table 1.1. Some are listed as normal changes because they have

Table 1.1. Frequently Occurring Changes with Advancing Age

BIOLOGICAL (universal) (Leventhal & Burns, 2004)	PSYCHOLOGICAL (Birren & Schaie, 2001; Rubert, Lowenstein, & Eisdorfer, 2004)
Decrease in stature	Slower in cognitive processing, reaction time
Up to 80% decrease in overall muscle mass	Eccentricites (sometimes cultural, sometimes typical for a generation, such as baby-boomer traits, called "cohort related"
Average 35% increase in total body fat (easier to gain weight)	
Skin atrophy (thinning, loss of subcutaneous fat, wrinkling)	Inappropriate self-disclosure (disinhibition)
Cataracts (90% by age 90)	Reduced risk taking (compared to youth)
Presbyacousia (loss of high tone hearing; can't hear consonants such as s, z, sh, ch, making speech less intelligible)	Continuity in behavioral patterns and personality
Presbyopia (loss of lens elasticity and accommodation for near vision)	Loss of stereotypic gender role association (e.g., men less aggressive, women more assertive)
Thickening of ventricular myocardium (decreased cardiac output)	Maintained sexual interest (though decreased performance)
Respiratory system changes (less elasticity, muscle atrophy, collagen rearrangement, decreased ciliary function—causes decreased vital capacity and less ventilatory volume)	Rigidity (controversial)* Disengagement (controversial)* Motivation shift to need for relatedness, autonomy, competence, rather than external goals (e.g., money, fame, good looks)
Circadian sleep timing change (sleep phase advances, decreased stages 3 and 4 sleep)	Reexamination of goals and attitudes Higher life satisfaction overall Recognition of mortality
Dental wear and gum reduction	
Gastric atrophy (decreased acid secretory capacity)	
Decreased myelin in cortex	
Decreased immune function (shift in leukocyte cell populations, impaired IL-2 production, possible decrease in cell function)	*Still, many elderly remain resilient and engaged, fitting the "older and wiser" stereotype.*
Decreased renal perfusion (glomerular filtration rate (GFR), decreased clearance)	
Menopause and atrophy of ovaries, breasts, and genitalia	
Decrease in testosterone; less atrophy than that of females	
Decreased sexual performance (erection, time to orgasm, etc., but often maintained sexual interest)	

SOCIAL (Birren & Schaie, 2001)	COGNITIVE (Birren & Schaie, 2001; Rubert et al., 2004; Leventhal, 2004)
Becoming a grandparent Death of parents and friends Retirement Increased wealth (savings, higher salaries if working)	Age-associated decline (1 standard deviation from the mean of younger people on a standardized memory test) Decline on digit symbol, letter comparison, pattern comparison, letter rotation, digit span, reading span, cued and free recall Maintenance of overall vocabulary and synonym and antonym vocabulary

not yet reached a point where they cause disability or warrant medical treatment. These changes nevertheless alter the elderly patient's resilience; medication tolerance, dosing (due to altered absorption), distribution, and metabolism (discussed later); flexibility; and, to some extent, self-expectations and behaviors.

Normal changes can also be positive, not just an indication of decline. Such normal improvements are usually visible in psychosocial domains. Consider the following:

- A decline in hostility and aggression occurs for most older adults (Cohen, 2005). The mellowing effect of age may be related to changes in neuronal circuits that cause blunted and less intense affect and less sustained emotional reactivity.
- Older adults are not as sensitive to social pressure based on what others might think of them; some use to full advantage the expectation that they will be outspoken and even inappropriate.
- Wisdom is also thought to come with age, and indeed there may be biological evidence that thinking is qualitatively different in older adults. In PET (positron emission tomography) studies, right and left brain are both active during problem solving in older adults, unlike younger brains that primarily use the dominant (reasoning) hemisphere. This bihemispheric processing with age may account for the ability to synthesize logic and feelings in decision making (Cabeza, 2002).
- Creativity is not often recognized in the elderly, but exists. Many authors and artists did some of their most famous works after age 60, such as Henri Matisse's design of the stained glass for the Dominican Chapel at Venice (age 82), Thomas Hobbes's *The Leviathan* (age 63), Katherine Graham's Pulitzer Prize for her autobiography (age 79), and countless other examples (Cohen, 2000). Common areas of creative change, if defined as any innovative positive life change, includes deepening relationships, revising roles (not a loss), creating a second life after retirement, responding to adversity with a new direction, or teaching what one has learned. Quoting from Cohen's (2000) book, Somerset Maugham stated: "When I was young I was amazed to learn

that the elder Cato [a Roman statesman] began at the age of 80 to learn Greek. I am amazed no longer. Old age is ready to undertake tasks that youth shirked because they would take too long."

Table 1.2. Normal versus Abnormal Changes Related to Aging

COMMON CHANGES Probably Normal	UNCOMMON CHANGES Probably Abnormal
1. Inappropriate self-disclosure (being more outspoken)	1. Disinhibition
2. Complaints about memory (metamemory)	2. Affective lability
3. Mild hypochondriacal concerns	3. Disorientation and new learning deficits
4. Hypervigilance (e.g., fear of falling, concerns about minor pains)	4. Excessive dependency (calls for help)
5. Slower retrieval of memories	5. Fear of being alone
6. Overinclusive thinking	6. Anxiety or panic
7. Tangential, storytelling style of speech	7. Prompts and cues don't help memory (processing speed)
8. Difficulty reaching main point (regional and cultural differences exist)	8. Does not recognize categorical differences
9. Fear of victimization ("cultural paranoia")	9. Social isolation and withdrawal

ANTI-AGING APPROACHES

Normal aging includes the concept of acceptance of death as part of the natural order. However, this acceptance runs against our societal phobia of aging. Prevention of aging has two definitions: One definition is finding immortality, the other, living a good quality of life until death. Even with healthy aging, there is, of course, a finite limit to the lifespan. The National Institute on Aging's (NIA) Long-Life Family Study (LLFS) reported that family longevity is an important predictor of a long life, but not as important as a positive mental attitude and health (www.longlife-familystudy.wustl.edu/LLFS/MessageNIA.html). (A longevity calculator from this study is available at www.livingto100.com). An analysis by Fries (1980) showed that if a survival curve were drawn (percent surviving on the *y*-axis and age on the *x*-axis), the plot would look increasingly like a rectangle, a so-called rectangular survival curve. People could live healthy, disease-free lives until the natural endpoint of life, when a terminal decline in the function of all organ systems occurs, usually in the year or so before death. Even in tissue cultures, cells stop dividing after a certain number of cell divisions (called the "Hayflick limit" [Hayflick, 1965]).

The term *anti-aging* usually refers to disease cessation and reduction of negative physical and cognitive decline. The lay press is replete with reports for DHEA (dehyroepiandrosterone), a natural steroid (adrenal, gonads, brain) that is converted to androstenedione, testosterone, and estrogen, as an anti-aging compound. DHEA is considered a dietary supplement by the Federal Drug Administration (FDA) and is available over the counter, whereas the actual hormonal treatment must be given by a physician. There is still no evidence that testosterone patches or DHEA or other hormones "retard aging" (Grimley, Malouf, Huppert, & van Niekerk, 2006). Growth hormone (GH) or dietary supplements that presumably increase GH secretion have also been touted in the literature, but still lack validation.

A more common and presumably safer intervention is the use of antioxidants. These agents prevent cellular damage from reactive oxygen species (i.e., free radicals) that form when unsaturated fatty acids are metabolized. Free radicals include hydrogen peroxide (H_2O_2), superoxide anion (O_2), and hydroxyl radical (-OH). Antioxidants also have minimal scientific evidence of efficacy but seem to cause no harm when used in moderation (see Table 1.3).

Table 1.3. Dietary Antioxidants

Vitamin A
Vitamin C
Vitamin E
Oxalic acid (cocoa/chocolate, spinach, berries)
Phytic acid (whole grains, maize)
Tannins (tea)

Source: From Fugh-Berman (2005); Flaherty & Morley (2004).

Although it is the least popular choice, calorie restriction and exercise are probably the most effective anti-aging interventions. For most people, this choice requires caloric monitoring, weight loss, and regular exercise. The ideal is to maintain a body mass index (BMI) in the normal range of 18.5–24. BMI is based on weight and height. A BMI table from the National Heart, Lung, & Blood Institute can be found in Appendix 1. The food pyramid still provides the optimal dietary plan. The U.S. Department of Agriculture lists 12 different plans on its website (www.mypyramid.gov). An example of a dietary worksheet from this government website can also be found in the appendix. Basically, the adage of eating more plants than meats, and eating meats with no legs (fish) more than two legs (foul) more than four legs (red meat) holds. In 2005 the Alzheimer's Association started a "Maintain Your Brain" program that emphasizes health promotion as the main early prevention intervention for Alzheimer's.

DEFINING OLD AGE

The joking response to the older person who asks "When does old age begin?" is "One year older than you," knowing that the person wouldn't ask if he or she weren't defensive about age. The real answer is actually a complicated social question. The traditional definition of old age is based on chronological age. Since the turn of the century, this marker was based on the age of retirement (age 55 minimum, age 65 traditionally). The age of retirement is actually a legislative artifact based on an age for which the percent of the population would not cause an excessive pension payout (at the time, less than 3% of the population). However, this rubric does not reflect how people define old age in real life. A typical reason that an older person gives for not considering a move to a residential community is "I don't want to be with all of those old people." The more natural clinical definition of old age refers to functional age (when a chronic disease or dementia appears) or biological age (when normal physical processes begin to decline). Social scientists, in contrast, focus on emotional age (when certain attitudes develop or disappear) or social age (when relationships and social roles change).

In lay terms, aging is often divided into categories of "young-old," "old," and "old-old," to differentiate people along these social and biological domains. Those in the young-old category are vibrant, healthy older people, who may be seeking an alternative to their old jobs and routines, usually in their 60s and early 70s. Those in the old category are viewed as slowing down or having different social roles. Old-old individuals are frail and usually of very advanced age. It is common for a disease-free 90-year-old to be considered "old" but to feel "young." The normal old person is becoming someone who is chronologically old, whose social roles have changed (retired, children are grown, may be widowed), but who remains healthy and active.

COUNTERTRANSFERENCE

Health-care professionals have their own "schemas" about elderly patients and what constitutes a positive outcome to treatment. Countertransference, as currently defined, differs from the original definition of the term. In the original definition of countertransference the therapist's unconscious needs and conflicts are projected onto the patient and impair his or her judgment about the patient. Currently the term refers to any unconscious reaction to the patient that affects the practitioner's understanding or treatment. Signs of common countertransferential reactions to patients are listed in Table 1.4.

Table 1.4. Signs of Countertransferential Ageism

1. Infantalization (treating the patient as if he or she were a child)
2. Failure to establish a working relationship
3. Premature termination (the patient won't come back)
4. Wrong diagnosis (especially overdiagnosis of dementia)
5. Missed diagnosis (assumption that pathological changes are normal for age)
6. Anger with the patient or family when either complains about lack of progress
7. Talking to the informant and not the patient

Nontherapeutic behaviors by the therapist or physician, such as treating elderly patients differently than other patients and assuming that pathological changes are normal, are probable evidence of a countertransferential ageism. If there is a discrepancy between the patient's presentation and statements and an informant's observations or test results, clinical judgment must be applied to determine if the family or the patient is distorting information. Because late-life delusions are usually not bizarre, complaints about family members may reflect a paranoid delusion. Conversely, family complaints and excessive negative views about the older person may reflect anger or interpersonal conflicts.

CASE EXAMPLE

Dr. C, a psychiatric resident, was on call when asked to admit an 81-year-old patient with Alzheimer's disease for violent behavior preceded by almost continuous psychomotor agitation for several weeks in a nursing home. After a brief interview in which the patient could not relate a coherent history, and without any laboratory testing, the resident sent the patient back to the nursing home with orders for prn haloperidol and a chastisement of the director of the nursing home for "dumping" the patient on the hospital. He told the director that dementia patients do not belong in a psychiatric hospital under any circumstance. Dr. C aspired to be a child psychiatrist and had no interest or understanding in dementia or elderly individuals. This example of an unwillingness to view dementia as a psychiatric problem can cross over to other behavioral issues in the elderly as well if care providers have severe countertransference issues. This must be guarded against to avoid inappropriate diagnosis or treatment.

SUCCESSFUL AGING

Successful aging is defined by positive life satisfaction and continued good physical and mental health. A recent longitudinal study on aging defined successful aging in terms of good functioning in the following six areas (Valliant & Mukamal, 2001): (1) physician-assessed objective physical health (absence of irreversible disability),

(2) subjective physical health, (3) length of active life, (4) objective mental health, (5) subjective life satisfaction, and (6) mutual satisfaction in relationships (social supports). The good news is that successful aging was related to controllable lifestyle factors more so than to uncontrollable factors such as genetics (family longevity, family histories) or a negative developmental history. Table 1.5 summarizes the correlates of successful aging and the factors deemed not significant.

Table 1.5. Correlates of Successful Aging vs. Factors Found Not Significant

CORRELATES OF SUCCESSFUL AGING:
- Education
- A healthy lifestyle
- Close relationships
- Suppression (not complaining)
- Mature psychological defenses (positive mental attitude)

NOT SIGNIFICANT
- Parental social class (e.g., coming from a wealthy family)
- Warmth of childhood (parenting)
- Childhood temperament
- Ancestral longevity (good genes; not significant or only weakly significant)

Source: From Vaillant & Mukamal (2001).

LATE-LIFE PSYCHOSOCIAL DEVELOPMENT

Stage theories mark "normal changes" in attitudes and behaviors related to sexuality, educational transitions, cognitive development, creativity, career, and family. The most widely accepted psychosocial theory is Eric Erikson's eight stages of human development (1963). Each stage represents a set of developmental tasks that involve psychological resolution of two opposing poles. Each task might be considered a dialectical dilemma in which a thesis and antithesis seek a synthesis. For example, the first stage of "trust versus mistrust" is usually best resolved by learning to give trust selectively, that is, neither trusting nor distrusting everyone. The eighth stage involves the issue of "integrity versus despair," wherein one must accept one's limitations and failings while still experiencing life as meaningful to self and others. A positive outcome in this stage is feeling that one has accomplished something and left a positive legacy that at least family will remember. What helps resolve a developmental crisis in old age is generally a life review that focuses on what was learned from both positive and negative life experiences and allows one to move on. Past stages, believed to be mastered, such as trust versus mistrust or industry versus inferiority, may also be revived. Table 1.6 summarizes Erikson's developmental model.

Table 1.6. Erikson's Eight Stages of Development

Stage 1 Trust versus mistrust
Stage 2 Autonomy versus shame and doubt
Stage 3 Initiative versus guilt
Stage 4 Industry versus inferiority
Stage 5 Identity versus identity diffusion
Stage 6 Industry versus isolation (first adult task)
Stage 7 Generativity versus self-absorption (second adult task—work, play, family)
Stage 8 Integrity versus despair (final adult task—meaning of life)

Source: From Erikson (1963).

Late-life development has also been viewed from other perspectives. Consider Colarusso and Nemiroff's lists of common issues and tasks in late life in Tables 1.7 and 1.8.

Table 1.7. Late-Life Adult Developmental Issues

1. Intimacy, love, and sex
2. The body
3. Time and death
4. Relationship to children
5. Relationship to parents
6. Mentor relationship
7. Relationship to society
8. Work
9. Play
10. Finances

Source: From Colarusso & Nemiroff (1987).

Table 1.8. Late-Life Adult Developmental Tasks

1. The aging process (chronic physical illness and health disability, the distinction being that chronic illness, like hypertension, diabetes, or arthritis, may not be disabling, whereas health disabilities are at the extreme end where function is impaired)
2. Illness or death of a loved one
3. Increased awareness of time limitation and one's own mortality (often consciousness is raised by diagnosis of a chronic medical condition such as hypertension, even if not disabling)
4. Changes in relationships with loved ones (if negative change)
5. A maturing spouse (drifted apart, personality changes, caregiving)
6. Recognition that all personal goals will not be reached (integrity vs. despair)
7. Planning for retirement

Source: From Colarusso & Nemiroff (1987).

Change can be out-of-synch from what the individual expects within any developmental stage. Stage theories suggest the appropriate clinical focus if the experience is not normative (i.e., not on the chart), is unexpected (novel), negative, life-threatening to self or loved ones, or life-changing (e.g., retirement, role changes).

CASE EXAMPLE

Mr. J is a 67-year old man who had been in excellent health throughout life and whose friends were all middle-aged coworkers in their 40s. He became depressed when forced to take early retirement, and at the same time he experienced his first chronic illness, hypertension. Even though his chronic illness was not disabling and he had a good pension, the changes were abrupt and outside of the expectation of his reference group. He also complained that his wife was becoming intolerable, seeming to have a change in personality and becoming more like his domineering mother who he could not wait to leave. These types of situations—changes that are out-of-synch with one's reference group expectations, revivals of old conflicts that one thought had been overcome, and chronic illness rather than losses or disability per se—are often the source of problems in older individuals.

There are no universal developmental milestones for old age. In children and adolescence a fairly predictable sequence of biological and intellectual growth and development (maturation) defines what can be expected when formal thinking, in Piaget's terms, develops, as well as social expectations. The standardized sequencing of school curricula and expectations seem more closely related to the actual developmental capacities of children than to some ideal progression of content. If children do not fit developmental expectations, they receive counseling or special classes. The situation is more complicated for adults, for whom expectations are largely socially determined by their reference group.

GROUP AND CULTURAL INFLUENCES

That groups exert power over individual behavior and attitudes is a well-accepted fact. As adults, individuals may find new reference groups as their models of behavior, but usually choose to maintain ties with the family of origin and the ethnic group with which they were raised. Examples of a reference group are racial or cultural (e.g., African American, Asian, Cajun, Mexican), geographical (e.g., Southerner, Northerner, Easterner, Californian), gender-related (e.g., gay, lesbian), or neighborhood-based (e.g., city, region). The behavioral and attitudinal prescriptions we absorb from our reference groups have been called "cognitive schemas." All schemas of adult development focus on the preferred patterns of how to cope with expectable illness, social role changes, decline, and loss. To fully appreciate the impact of this dynamic, it is useful for psychiatrists to have a broad knowledge of sociology, psychology, and different cultures. Intuition improves with clinical experience as professionals gain knowledge of social science, developmental theory, reference group theory, psychosocial development, and cultural perspectives. Intuition, after all, is little more than making correct inferences when direct information is lacking (i.e., an educated guess).

A culturally sensitive approach to psychiatry tries to reintegrate the patient into their reference group or social network, unless that group is clearly pathological or destructive. The approach also tries to establish whether the patient's expectations of what should be happening at his or her age are "off track" in light of their social norms, and helps reestablish a sense of control and expectability.

Culture, in particular, often provides the reference group and rules that one uses to judge "normalcy" or what is right. "Middle-class values" may not be considered "normal" to other groups. In fact, some may label such values prudish, obsessional, or inhibited. To a teen culture, old age begins at 30—people over 30 are "ancient ones." "Acting one's age" is often a cultural definition, as is a "normal relationship" with one's children. For example, family-centered cultures such as Hispanic or Asian may expect a daughter to give up work to care for the aging parent, or to have the parent move in with her. Treatment preferences also seem to be culturally defined, and are obviously strongest in groups that have been neither acculturated (e.g., immigrants) or assimilated (ostracism due to prejudice).

A common misconception among professionals is that cultural sensitivity means applying alternative medicine practices. This cannot be further from the truth. Cultural sensitivity means understanding the patient's frame of reference about illness and aging. Key issues include (1) beliefs that some illnesses are normal, (2) fear of prejudice, (3) what constitutes normative experiences, (4) views on aging, (5) various communication barriers, and (6) differences in nonverbal cues. Cultural barriers often seem to disappear once trust is gained. The following points are key elements in providing culturally sensitive care:

- Consider noncompliance from a minority patient as a potential cultural difference.
- Confront suspected cultural differences early and establish a compromise position only if the issue interferes with the relationship or treatment.
- View the cultural issue as if it were a negative transference issue (barrier to work).
- Be especially cognizant of the policy of "minimal intervention"—for example, house the elderly patient in the least restrictive environment (avoid nursing homes).

Table 1.9 summarizes the types of culturally influenced issues and areas of which practitioners should be aware.

Table 1.9. Culturally Influenced Areas and Issues

Language barriers
Trust in "Western medical practices"
Attitude toward psychiatry
Views of causality of illness (e.g., folk beliefs)
Treatment preferences (e.g., attitude toward medications, folk cures)
Definition of old age
Behavioral norms for an old person
Signs of respect or deference
Health locus of control (i.e., what they do can make a difference, versus relying
   on the doctor or fate)
Socioeconomic status (effect of prejudicial treatment and opportunities)
Resource availability
Family size and involvement (children's roles, caregiving)
Willingness to accept outside help
Attitudes toward nursing homes

BIOPSYCHOSOCIAL MODEL

The biopsychosocial model lies at the center of geriatric practice. This model emphasizes the importance of exploring and treating interacting biological and medical factors (predisposition), psychological factors (appraisal style and coping skills), and social factors (economics, social support, stress) at the same time. Generally, the biopsychosocial view is that a patient with a predisposition (due to a genetic or developmental factor) who is overwhelmed by stress (negative environmental events) is likely to develop a psychiatric illness. Social features such as family, friends, and resources may be a source of stress or may act as a buffer to help the person cope with the stress. Once an illness begins, it may develop its own intrinsic "rhythm," whereby recurrences are no longer clearly linked to stress, or may recur with milder stress.

A similar view is the concept of allostasis (McEwen & Wingfield, 2003). Individuals must adjust their physiology, morphology, and behavior to changing environments—that is, maintaining stability through change, or adaptation. The concept of homeostasis does not capture this dynamic and ever-changing balance. When the changing environment cannot be adapted to, allostatic overload occurs, and eventually irreversible negative changes may become manifest.

Solutions to allostatic overload and to breakdowns in the biopsychosocial model are similar. Intervention can (1) teach patients to recognize stressful situations earlier and either withdraw, learn better coping skills, or respond differently through psychotherapy; (2) address biological aspects (medications or other biological treatments); (3) increase social supports (buffers); or (4) remove stressors. Intervening at any level may be sufficient to achieve remission, but intervening at all levels is logically the best approach. An example of this need to intervene on all levels is an extreme reaction to a loss or separation. It is clearly the patient's appraisal of the meaning of the loss that causes pathological mourning and excessive psychiatric reactions (Bowlby, 1980), and that appraisal would need to be addressed in psychotherapy. Fear may lead to a catastrophic reaction even if the stress is relatively minimal.

George Pollock, the former head of the Psychoanalytic Institute in Chicago and past president of the American Psychiatric Association (1983–84), created an equation (unpublished) he called Pollock's "3-P's" to encompass the biopsychosocial approach:

Predisposition + Precipitating Event(s) + Perpetuating Circumstances − Buffers = Outcome

Predispositions are biological factors (strong familial histories or developmental experiences such as trauma or abuse). *Precipitating events* are stressors (loss of job, divorce) that are influenced by appraisal. *Perpetuating circumstances* are chronic sources of stress that prevent one from getting well, and *buffers* are sources of help, such as family support, coping skills, and appraisal strengths. Treatment of predispositions involves medication and psychotherapy. Psychotherapy can help patients gain insight, learn better coping mechanisms, and feel more in control of their lives. The changes practitioners initiate, such as restoring the supportive network or other social interventions (e.g., housing or financial aid) may help redress "perpetuating factors." Table 1.10 summarizes the components of Pollock's "3-P's."

Table 1.10. Pollock's Biopsychosocial Components

PREDISPOSITION	PRECIPITATING EVENT(S)	PERPETUATING CIRCUMSTANCES	BUFFERS
Family history (genetic loading)	Illness, disability	Chaotic family	Strong family support
Developmental events	Loss	High emotionality	Coping skills
Early parent loss	Retirement	Low socioeco- nomic level	Appraisal style
Parental warmth	Cumulative stress		
Prior episodes	Relocation		

This formula reflects the areas that need to be addressed in treatment. Medications alone to handle genetic predispositions and biological changes are usually not enough to shift the balance of the equation to health. Psychotherapy to improve coping or understanding, or psychosocial interventions to reduce environmental stress or improve the supportive network are usually needed.

COMMON PSYCHIATRIC DISORDERS

The most common psychiatric problems seen in elderly populations are listed in Table 1.11. Actual rates are not given here because the methodologies vary so much from study to study. Some studies have relatively small numbers of subjects, and most use different measurement instruments or figures that are based on so-called convenience samples of patients who present spontaneously for care at clinics or hospitals. The last epidemiological catchment area survey by the National Institute of Mental Health (NIMH) was completed in 1982.

It is important to impress upon medical colleagues that screening is needed and is not time consuming—it is part of following up on clinical impressions. Often the response to a single question such as "Do you feel depressed?" is enough to determine if further probing is needed. It is also important to screen for potential iatrogenic or medication-induced side effects, which often mimic psychiatric problems. Patients should bring in their current medications and vitamins periodically and inform whenever any new over-the-counter or prescription medication is started.

Table 1.11. Psychiatric Conditions Commonly
Encountered in Older Adults

MOST COMMON
Pathological grief (defined by severity or duration > 6 months)
Depression (often with mood-congruent delusions, nihilism, factitious illness)
Anxiety
Suicide risk (highest with depression, alcohol abuse, psychosis [due to
    impulsivity])
Dementia with behavioral disturbance
Delirium
Somatization complaints (usually do not meet full DSM critiera)
Psychosomatic problems (illness caused by emotional problems)
Medication misuse

LESS COMMON
Bipolar disorder
Obsessive–compulsive disorder (OCD)
Schizophrenia (occasionally late onset; paraphrenia)
Borderline personality disorder
Substance abuse
Partial complex seizure disorder

Source: From Gurland (2004); NAMI NH (2001).

Of particular note, 14% of elderly patients develop a major depression within 2 years of the loss of a spouse or child (AAGP, 2004). About 10% of elderly patients show phobias (e.g., safety fears and fear of leaving their home), and phobias are present in over 40% of other psychiatric disorders. The rate of suicide is more than five times higher in white men over age 85 (50/100,000) but still high in elderly white women (12/100,000) (AAGP, 2001). The rate of behavioral disturbances in patients with dementia exceeds 50% (Mega, Cummings, Fiorello & Gornbein, 1896). Delirium occurs in over 30% of hospitalized patients (when studies are conducted) but is recognized in less than 3% (what is typically charted) (Levkoft, Evans, Liptzin, et al., 1991).

Older patients are often more motivated for treatment than younger patients, if a therapeutic alliance is achieved. They often have better social skills, ego strengths, and experiences with which to facilitate change. The practitioner sees less acting out, manipulation, or violence in geriatric patients. On the other hand, the need to accommodate mild cognitive impairment, sensory impairment, communication problems, and slower cognitive speed of processing often complicates treatment. In the next chapter we examine the salient clinical considerations involved in geriatric psychopharmacology.

SUMMARY

Our current demographic situation makes it imperative that we pay attention to our older adults. Many of the negative stereotypes about aging are due to the expectation of illness and disability with age. Although illness is common, it is never "normal" to be sick as one gets older. This applies to dementia and depression as well as to physical diseases. Understanding the difference between "normal" and "abnormal" changes common to aging is crucial, as is recognizing the importance of a more practical definition of the biopsychosocial model.

2

GERIATRIC PSYCHOPHARMACOLOGY:
CLINICAL CONSIDERATIONS

This chapter provides an overview of the general principles and guidelines involved in prescribing medication for older adults. (Specific medications and protocols for agitation in dementia, depression, psychosis, anxiety, and sleep are addressed in subsequent chapters.) Clinicians often ask "What medication is best for [choose disorder] in the elderly?" "What is the optimal dose to use?" "Are the risks different?" Psychopharmacology for geriatric patients requires close attention to basic pharmacology principles because of changes in pharmacokinetics, drug interactions, and "end organ sensitivity." The major reasons for altering prescribing practices for patients of advanced age are:

- Psychotropic drug metabolism changes (slower metabolism for a variety of reasons).
- Volume of distribution changes (more fat stores).
- Free medication level is often higher (less total body water and nutritional deficiencies may alter blood carrier proteins such as albumin).
- Medication interactions are more likely (the average old-old person is on eight medications).
- Older adults are frailer and more prone to injury from medication side effects.

EVIDENCE-BASED PRACTICE IN PSYCHOPHARMACOLOGY

Given the potential of lawsuits for inappropriate treatment, even in the absence of damages, it is becoming increasingly important to utilize evidence-based medicine when prescribing any medication to geriatric patients. Many reviews employ a system for evaluating the quality of evidence, shown in Table 2.1. The Cochrane Reviews (www.cochrane.com) look for Class I evidence and Level A recommendations. Off-label uses of medications usually fit Level C or D (low evidence base), and most augmentation strategies used in clinical practice usually fit Level D (clinical opinion only).

Table 2.1. Categories of Evidence and
Levels of Recommendation

CATEGORIES OF EVIDENCE

Class I: From one or more randomized, controlled trials (or meta-analysis)

Class II: From at least one controlled study without randomization or other type of quasi-experimental study

Class III: From a nonexperimental study (comparative studies, correlation studies, or case-controlled studies)

Class IV: From committee reports or opinions and/or clinical experience of respected authorities

STRENGTH OF RECOMMENDATIONS

Level A: Directly based on Class I evidence

Level B: Directly based on Class II evidence or extrapolated from Class I evidence

Level C: Directly based on Class III evidence or extrapolated from Class I or II evidence

Level D: Directly based on Class IV evidence or extrapolated from Class I, II, or III evidence

---

Class I or II evidence is preferred but is often not available for elderly patients. Data from healthy general adult populations are typically used for all age groups but are not reliable for special populations such as frail older adults or patients on concomitant medications.

In general, case reports (Class III data) should be used cautiously. Usually 80% of case reports are positive for the medication discussed because people are more likely to report their successes than failures (the Pollyanna principle). If the number of positive case reports is lower than 60%, it is thought to be nonrobust—that is, too low to pursue in a large placebo-controlled clinical trial. Open-label studies with larger numbers of subjects show a similar propensity for a positive response bias (the investigator wants to prove his or her idea and interprets data through "rose-colored glasses"), although to a lesser degree than case reports. These factors explain why it is so important to read studies carefully and compare the population in the study to the patient you are treating for similarities in dosing needs and expected speed of response.

There is one problem with evidence-based practice in relation to elderly patients: data are often limited to younger adult patients. Additionally, psychotropic medication use in elderly patients is often off-label. For example, it is not a far stretch of the imagination to think that psychosis associated with delirium or dementia may be treated with antipsychotics, even though approval of antipsychotics is limited to schizophrenia and bipolar mania (later chapters, however, show that this issue is a little more complicated).

Optimal dosing in older adults is also far from certain. Geriatrics, more than general adult psychiatry, requires attention to preclinical data on kinetics, protein binding, metabolism, and excretion to provide a rationale for dose adjustments in special conditions.

In addition to off-label prescribing decisions and lack of information on dosing, practitioners often lament that "clinical trials are nothing like clinical practice." This is true in that clinical practice involves more comorbid medical conditions, potentially worse compliance, and use of concomitant medications that are not allowed in clinical trials.

These additional conditions make it all the more important to use clinical trial data as the starting point and use preclinical data of pharmacokinetics, adverse effects, and receptor profiles to adjust medication doses. That is, clinical trials provide information about treatment *under optimal conditions*. It is up to the clinician to make the needed adjustments to compensate for medical comorbidity, frailty, concomitant medications, and the metabolic abnormalities that many elderly people show.

When assessing clinical trials for a particular medication, ask yourself the following questions:

- Are the patients included in the trial similar to my patient, other than age?

- How much was safe (dose range)?
- How fast was improvement seen (speed of response)?
- What were the main side effects?

Expanded review criteria are provided in Table 2.2.

Table 2.2. Review Criteria for Evaluating Clinical Trials of Medications

Inclusion and exclusion criteria	Similar population other than age? What were the health restrictions (exclusion criteria) and why?
Scales used	What target symptoms were followed?
Speed of response	When did improvement begin? (e.g., 2-week point)
Rate of remission	What was the rate of remission by the end of the study? What percent had improved (e.g., 50% reduction in scale score)?
Doses	What was the maximally effective dose? Did adverse events go up markedly with higher doses? Is once-daily or split dosing needed?
Secondary symptoms	Did the medication also reduce anxiety or somatic complaints, or improve sleep?
Safety versus side effects	What adverse effects occurred at what dose? What was the early termination rate (often a mark of the clinical importance of the side effect)?
Placebo response	What was the true effect of the medication or true rate of adverse effects (what occurred above the placebo level)?
Rescue medication	What is the best medication to relieve symptoms while doing dose titration or waiting for clinical effect? (Often studies allow a tranquilizer during the early phase of a trial.)

GERIATRIC PRESCRIBING CONSIDERATIONS

If one were to ask for a printout of potential drug interactions from the hospital pharmacy regarding an inpatient, there would be greater than a 90% likelihood of some drug interaction if the patient is on three or more medications. The only practical way to minimize adverse effects in elderly patients and still find the minimum effective dose is to apply the following geriatric prescribing rules:

1. Start low, go slow (titrate slowly), but go (titrate to the lower of the maximum tolerated dose or highest recommended dose).
2. Avoid polypharmacy.
3. Avoid augmentation.
4. Use sequential single medication trials for medication failures, going to a medication from a different class rather than another medication from the same class. For example, if an SSRI (selective serotonin reuptake inhibitor) fails, switch to an SNRI (serotonin-norepinephrine reuptake inhibitor) next.

CASE EXAMPLE

Ms. J is a 72-year-old woman with a long history of schizophrenia. She was appropriately switched from 24 mg bid perphenazine to 0.5 mg qd risperidone when tardive dyskinesia developed, but the dose was never adjusted to clinical response. She relapsed within months and moved to another city to be closer to her children who could help monitor her care. The children had their mother admitted to a psychiatric hospital when she became paranoid and threatening (thinking that her children were trying to poison her), socially withdrawn and preoccupied, and refused her medications. When admitted to a general psychiatry unit, she was started on citalopram for depression and was kept on risperidone, but was also started on olanzepine for psychosis, haloperidol prn for aggression, clonazepam for sleep, and donepazil for confusion. The patient was mildly obese with controlled adult-onset non-insulin-dependent diabetes, hypertension, and arthritis. Her confusion and difficulty concentrating reportedly occurred during the hospitalization. Upon discharge, the family sought consultation from geriatric psychiatry because the patient seemed "drugged and confused" and the cost of medications was not affordable.

In this case, it was very reasonable to change to an atypical antipsychotic because of the emergence of tardive dyskinesia. However, equivalent doses should be used or titrated to reestablish the new, optimal dose. In this case there was no reason to start multiple antipsychotics and benzodiazepines during the hospitalization. Polypharmacy only caused cognitive impairment and gait disturbance. Olanzepine and certain psychotropics are also ill advised as initial choices in patients with diabetes and obesity. Furthermore, using Alzheimer's medications to treat the cognitive side effects of psychotropic medications is also ill advised.

SELECTION: WHICH MEDICATION IS BEST?

Specific studies regarding efficacy, dosing, and adverse effects are often lacking for elderly populations, and almost *always* lacking for frail elderly with comorbid diseases. In the absence of research-based decisions, *medication selection* should follow these geriatric prescribing rules:

1. Choose medications for specific target symptoms.
2. Select between medications by desired side effects (e.g., sedation vs. activation).
3. Avoid medications by undesired side effects (e.g., avoid medications that cause diabetes or obesity in patients with preexisting problems in that area; avoid medications that cause hypertension or hypotension when a patient already has that health problem).
4. Change medications rather than using megadoses of an ineffective medication (more is not better).
5. Change the medication before using augmentation strategies if a medication is ineffective (sequential single medication trials are preferred).
6. Use electroconvulsive therapy (ECT) after two adequate antidepressant trials.
7. Add psychotherapy.

No reliable predictor of the best starting medication currently exists. In the future, medications may be chosen based on genetic subtyping. Generally, we still use common-sense rules for selecting medications, often choosing the first medication based on desirable side effects, such as a propensity for sedation, versus side effects to avoid due to comorbid medical conditions. For example, a depressed elderly patient with many concomitant medications who complains of anergy can be started on citalopram (a generic SSRI), which has little sedation and does not utilize 2D6 or 3A4 CYP450 as its primary metabolic pathway. These enzymes are involved in the metabolism of more than 60% of existing medications. Similarly, a geriatric patient with significant anxiety, agitation, and insomnia may do better with a more sedating SSRI such as paroxetine (a generic SSRI) or trazadone (another generic medication) at bedtime.

Patients suffering from side effects often improve when clinicians eliminate multiple medications, reduce doses, or are more thoughtful about medication selection. One geriatrician's definition of his role was "A geriatrician is the doctor who stops the drugs other doctor's start." It is usually preferable to change a medication rather than treat a side effect with a second medication. For example, if extrapyramidal symptoms are observed from an antipsychotic, switch antipsychotics instead of adding an anticholinergic medication—especially given the plethora of medication choices now that was not present a few decades ago.

A more scientific approach is to use receptor affinity tables as potential predictors of response and side effects. In this type of calculation, K_i is the affinity constant for an antipsychotic receptor. This K_i value is actually roughly equivalent to the concentration in nanamoles (nM) that shows equivalent binding to 1 nM of the parent compound, such as acetylcholine at muscarinic receptors (M_1), dopamine at D_1 or D_2 receptors, serotonin (5-HT), histamine (H_1), or norepinephrine receptors (α_1-adrenergic). A value of less than 1 means that the medication binds more readily than the comparator, so it would take less than 1 nM concentration to bind to as many receptors as 1 nM of the parent compound. A value of more than 1 means that the medication would take a higher concentration to bind as readily as 1 nM of the parent compound.

The K_i tables (Richelman, 1999, 2001, 2003) are often misinterpreted. Put as simply as possible, a high affinity medication

($K_i<1$) will require a low milligram dosing (1 milligram or more), and a low affinity medication ($K_i>1$) will require a high milligram dosing (100 milligrams or more). Any other receptor with a K_i value of at least a 1:10 ratio is likely to be close enough to have a clinical effect at that receptor. In the absence of direct clinical data, these K_i tables help to determine which psychotropic drugs might cause a specific adverse effect as the dose is pushed higher, meaning any drug that approaches a 1:10 ratio to the target receptor. (A good discussion of pharmacokinetic modeling is given in Greenblatt et al., 2000.) Table 2.3 provides a profile of K_i values for antipsychotic drugs.

Table 2.3. Receptor-Binding Profile of Antipsychotics (K_i Values)

	Aripiprazole	Olanzapine	Risperidone	Quetiapine	Ziprasidone	Clozapine	Haloperiodol
D_2	0.34	11	3	160	4.8	125	1
$5\text{-}HT_{2A}$	3.4	4	0.6	220	0.4	12	78
$5\text{-}HT_{2C}$	15	11	26	615	1.3	8	3085
α_1	57	19	2	7	10	7	46
H_1	61	7	155	11	47	6	3630
M_1	>10,000	1.9	> 5000	120	>10,000	1.9	1,475

Note. K_i is a constant indexed to reflect relative binding in comparison to 1 nM of the target compound (e.g., 1 nM of dopamine at the D_2 receptor has a $K_i = 1$). Lower number means higher potency, unlike K_d value below. Adapted from information slide from Bristol-Myers Squibb (2002) and Richelson (1999). Code: D = dopamine; 5-HT = 5 hydroxytryptophan (serotonin); α = α-adrenergic; H = histamine; M = muscarinic.

Typical antipsychotic doses were found to have clinical efficacy between 60 and 80% D_2 receptor blockade. For a medication such as aripiprazole, the table shows that it would take >10,000 nM of aripiprazole to have the same binding as 1 nM of acetylcholine at the M_1 receptor. If it takes 0.34 nM of aripiprazole to have as much binding as 1 nM of dopamine at the D_2 receptor, it is not hard to see that a therapeutic concentration (at the D_2 receptor) would have a negligible effect on muscarinic receptors. From Table 2.3, one would expect significant serotonin reuptake inhibition at doses leading to therapeutic effects when the ratio of D_2 to $5\text{-}HT_2$ is about 1:10. Similarly, a ratio of 1:10 or lower for

D_2 with any other receptor is likely to have a significant clinical effect at the non-D_2 receptor showing that ratio.

Based on the table, one might expect more antidepressant and anxiolytic effects when the serotonin–dopamine ratio is low (closer in affinity), as in olanzapine, compared to the other novel antipsychotics. Many clinicians feel that this is true in their clinical experience. Similarly, one might expect less cognitive impairment when there is less blockade of muscarinic receptors. This information allows a rationale for initial medication selection, although it is still far from perfect. Table 2.4 provides a profile of K_d values for antidepressants. The K_d value reflects the equilibrium dissociation constant and is similar to K_i.

Table 2.4. Receptor-Binding Profile of Antidepressants (K_d Values)

	Mirtazapine	Citalopram	Fluoxetine	Duloxetine	Venlafaxine	Sertraline	Desipramine
D_2	0.001	0.003	0.028	0.12	0.01	4	0.03
5-HT_{2A}	0.001	90	120	NA	11	340	5.7
NE	0.021	0.025	0.41	NA	0.094	0.24	120
α_1	0.2	0.053	0.017	NA	0	0.27	0.77
H_1	700	0.2	0.02	0.04	0	0.004	0.9
M_1	0.15	0.045	0.05	0.033	0	0.16	0.5

Note. K_d is the equilibrium dissociation constant (similar to K_i; Richelson, 2001). Higher number means higher potency. Code: D = dopamine; 5-HT = 5 hydroxytryptophan (serotonin); NE = norepinephrine; a = alpha-adrenergic; H = histamine; M = muscarinic; NA = not available.

The target receptor for dosing in depression is 5-HT and/or norepinephrine (NE). If a medication's affinity at receptors other than 5-HT or NE is within 1/10th the potency, it probably will show a clinical effect at that receptor. As can be seen, most of the antidepressants noted in Table 2.4 should have minimal adverse effects—a prediction borne out at therapeutic doses. Other than cardiac effects, which are not predicted by any of the receptor affinities noted in Table 2.4, the main concern is with confusion (M_1) and blood pressure (α_1 and NE). Generally, SSRIs and newer medications provide little source of concern in these side effects, based on the tables, whereas tricyclic antidepressants

(TCAs) might. Thus TCAs would generally be a late choice in patients with dementia or orthostatic hypotension because of their affect on M_1 and α_1 receptors, as predicted from the tables. As with antipsychotics, the tables are mainly helpful in determining relative likelihood of producing a given side effect, as doses are increased (and some side effects may be beneficial, e.g., sedation at night).

What Preclinical Information is Useful?

The *Physician's Desk Reference* (PDR) usually contains enough information to make an educated guess about potential drug interactions and duration of drug action when evidence-based data or specific guidelines are not available. Table 2.5 summarizes the function of major pharmacokinetic parameters that may help determine medication selection.

Table 2.5. Functions of Major Pharmacokinetic Parameters

PARAMETER	FUNCTION
tmax (time to peak absorption)	Predicts time for maximum response if effects are related to blood levels.
$t_{1/2}$ (elimination half-life)	Predicts dosing frequency and steady state.
Protein binding (%)	For lipid-soluble medications, this is the main way medications are carried. For a 99% protein-bound medication, a 1% displacement from binding sites doubles the free drug level.
Metabolism	Predicts potential drug interactions of medications metabolized in the same way.
Excretion	Predicts how much is eliminated unchanged. Is the primary excretion hepatic or renal?

Hepatic Metabolism

Most medications are metabolized in the liver. It is widely accepted that the step that leads to oxidative hydroxylation, or deethylation, catalyzed by the P450 enzyme system (labeled

CYP450 for cytochrome P450), is usually the rate-limiting step of metabolism (i.e., the slowest part). The P450 system is comprised of about 60 enzymes clustered into different "families" based on molecular weight, the compounds they metabolize (substrate specificity), and spectral properties. These are divided further into isoenzymes, or genetic variations of each enzyme. Only a tiny difference in amino acid sequence is enough to change the enzyme's fit with different substrates and its effectiveness as a catalyst. There are two major classes of P450 enzymes: mitochondrial isoenzymes, which catalyze the formation of endogenous substances (steroids, prostaglandins, fatty acids), and those in the endoplasmic reticulum, which metabolize a large percentage of medications. The CYP450 enzymes can be induced by some medications, inhibited by others, or may have to metabolize multiple medications simultaneously, leading to competition for the same enzyme. At times, genetic variations or multiple forms of P450 subtypes may make the enzyme less or more effective. The net effect is that slow metabolism can result (slow metabolizers), leading to toxicity at lower doses of a medication, or fast metabolism can result (fast metabolizers), leading to ineffectiveness of a medication because the levels remain low.

Slower absorption, decreased cardiac output, reduced renal clearance, more fat relative to muscle, less total body water, and at times malnutrition all predict a need to lower doses. These factors are highly variable from individual to individual. CYP genetic profiling or detailed drug interaction charts are not routine, but because genetic subtyping of human CYP450 is now commercially available, it should be considered when a patient has an atypical response to medications, such as showing intolerance to extremely low doses of a medication or not responding to any medication. Drug interaction lists are readily available on the Internet and show which medications are metabolized by each CYP450, allowing one to avoid medications metabolized by a deficient CYP450, or medications that are all metabolized by the same CYP450. Ordinarily, competition for the same enzyme system requires only dose adjustments, not cessation of use of medications. Table 2.6 shows which P450 genes metabolize which psychotropic medications.

Table 2.6. Human P450 Genes Responsible for
Psychotropic Medication Metabolism

1A2 (Chromosome 15)	amitriptyline, clomipramine, clozapine, fluvoxamine, haloperidol, imipramine, olanzapine // warfarin, caffeine
2B6 (Chromosome 19)	bupropion, methadone
2C8 (Chromosome 10)	NA
2C9 (Chromosome 10)	amitriptyline, fluoxetine // most NSAIDS, warfarin, many sulfonylureas, losartan
2C19 (Chromosome 10)	diazepam, amitriptyline, citalopram, clomipramine // warfarin, phenytoin, hexobarbital, propranolol, many protein pump inhibitors
2D6 (Chromosome 22)	amitriptyline, clomipramine, desipramine, imipramine, paroxetine, haloperidol, perphenazine, risperidone, thioridazine, amphetamine, aripiprazole, duloxetine, fluoxetine, nortriptyline, venlafaxine // oxycodone, propranolol, quinidine
2E1 (Chromosome 10)	ethanol
3A4, 5, 7 (Chromosome 7)	alprazolam, diazepam, midazolam, triazolam // carbamazepine, steroids, many statins, many HIV antivirals, many calcium channel blockers, quinidine, chlorpheniramine, astemizole

Note. Medications following the double slash marks (//) represent common concomitant medications. NA = not applicable.

As an example, when prescribing fluoxetine and olanzapine together for depressive episodes of bipolar disorder, be aware that both are metabolized by 2D6 and may affect each other's metabolism. When the medications are combined in a combination (e.g., Symbyax) the dose of fluoxetine is reduced by 20%, but olanzapine remains unchanged. Similarly, when giving aripiprazole together with fluoxetine for the same indication, or if given with carbamazepine, the dose of aripiprazole is reduced 50%, but fluoxetine and carbamazepine doses remain unchanged. Practically speaking, there is no contraindication to using medications together as long as dose titration is slow and dosage increases are stopped when adverse effects first appear, rather than pushing to an projected dose.

Dosing Considerations

Once a medication is selected, the general strategy to set the appropriate dose can be summarized in Table 2.7.

Table 2.7. General Dosing Strategy

1. Start at $^1/_3$ to $^1/_2$ the usual starting dose.
2. Increase the dose rapidly to the target dose (unless clinical trials show better tolerance with slower titration; e.g., current AD medications).
3. Increase at about five half-life intervals (e.g., for medications with 24-hour half-lives, steady state is usually reached in 5–7 days).
4. Monitor target symptoms and adverse effects often (I advise weekly or at least every 2 weeks during dose titration phase).
5. If there is not about 50% improvement in target symptoms compared to baseline after at least a 2-week trial on the maximum dose, change to a different class of medication that is approved for the disorder (this is usually a 6- to 8-week trial overall).
6. If there is more than 50% improvement in target symptoms, maintain the same medication at the same dose; improvements usually continue to occur slowly.
7. If clinical improvement has reached a plateau but significant residual symptoms exist, consider augmentation to treat the residual symptoms.
8. During the titration phase, a hypnotic may be needed for sleep, or an additional medication may be needed for sedation, but this should be terminated later.

It should be common sense that using more than one medication from the same class of compounds (polypharmacy) and using doses that exceed the recommended range (supratherapeutic dosing) are not wise with any patient. In elderly patients this practice is especially dangerous. Consider the factors noted in Table 2.8.

Table 2.8. Pharmacokinetic Changes in the Elderly

1. Pharmacokinetic considerations
   a. Slower absorption
   b. Different volumes of distribution at steady state
   c. Lower cardiac output due to disease states (may slow delivery of blood to the liver and reduce renal clearance)
2. Potential drug interactions may occur when multiple medications are taken
3. Frailty (in the old-old) concomitants
   a. Higher risk for falls
   b. Higher risk for confusion
   c. Higher risk for cardiac side effects
   d. Higher risk for orthostatic hypotension
   e. Higher rates of medication side effects
4. Genetic polymorphisms of hepatic enzymes predict slow or rapid metabolism

The only exceptions apply to the following conditions:

- Higher than average dosing is acceptable if poor absorption or rapid metabolism is suspected (blood levels are helpful).
- Augmentation is acceptable if response to the first medication has been partial with only a residual symptom such as continued insomnia or anergy, but potential drug interactions should be considered.

MEDICATION TRIALS

Informed Consent for Medications

It is important to warn patients to watch for the most common or most dangerous side effects without scaring them. If side effects are minor, one can usually warn the patient in a matter-of-fact way. For example, anticholinergic properties of a medication may be presented by saying, "You will be close to the therapeutic dose when you begin to notice a little dryness in your mouth. Just keep sugarless candy in your mouth to keep the saliva flowing." Constipation can be addressed by saying "Take milk of magnesia a few times a week if you notice any constipation." The possibility of confusion can be addressed by saying

"Some people complain of slight confusion on this medication. This may go away within a few weeks, but even if it doesn't, most find it better not to stop if the medication is working. If you or I feel the confusion is making it difficult to function, we'll have to stop it."

What If the First Medication Trial Is Ineffective?

The first consideration when there is poor response to medication is to determine whether the patient is taking the appropriate dose. The next consideration is whether the diagnosis is correct.

The usual steps to take when a patient is not taking medications as prescribed are psychoeducation and setting up a system for supervision. Psychoeducation means explaining the importance of medications—what they do and their benefits and risks—and working out logistical problems of administration. For example, if a medication causes a dry mouth (xerostomia), the patient can be told that this is a minor, albeit annoying, side effect that can be handled by sucking on sugarless candy or gum or taking small sips of water throughout the day. It is always best to prescribe medications that can be administered once a day; even short half-life medications are available in extended-release preparations. Link medication administration to some habitual activity, such as when the patient goes to bed, eats, or wakes up in the morning. If cost is the issue, generics are essential unless specific health considerations or a differential response mandate use of newer medications with different side effect profiles. Supervision is the second way to improve compliance with medications. This method requires a reminder system, someone to fill pill containers and monitor them, or, at the far extreme, someone to administer the medication directly. Direct administration usually requires the availability and willingness of someone living in the household with the patient.

If a patient is not responding and compliance is confirmed, review the diagnostic criteria for use of the medication. Figure 2.1 presents a "decision tree" that can be helpful in sorting through the pros and cons of various options when medication has produced an undesirable (or no) response.

Figure 2.1. Clarifying the reason for medication nonresponse and identifying the next best step.

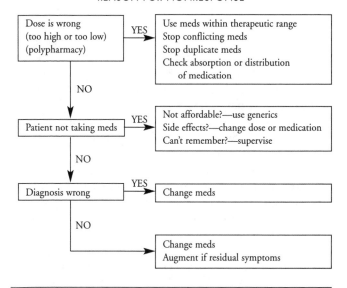

REASON FOR NONRESPONSE

Augmentation

Augmentation is the new term for polypharmacy. In most cases, augmentation is not advised with the elderly because of potential drug interactions that cause adverse effects. However, for any disorder, if there is a partial response to a medication it may be helpful to consider a second medication for residual symptoms. Common examples of a partial response with residual symptoms include treatment for depression or psychosis with problems of insomnia, hypersomnia, or generalized anxiety. In such cases, hypnotics may be prescribed to induce sleep, stimulants may be used to increase wakefulness, or benzodiazepines or novel antipsychotics may be added to reduce anxiety. Studies for augmentation for any disorder are usually at a Level C or D (not based on controlled studies). Typically, the following strategies are employed:

- Augment a novel antipsychotic at maximum tolerated dose with a typical antipsychotic at low dose to improve dopamine blockade for partial responders (e.g., quetiapine plus perphenazine).
- Augment an antidepressant with T3 or lithium (there is evidence of efficacy with this combination in younger patients).
- Augment an antidepressant with a novel antipsychotic, especially with mood-congruent delusions or other psychotic symptoms. (The reason to use a novel antipsychotic instead of a typical is mainly the risk of tardive dyskinesia, but typicals also have more dose-related side effects.)
- Use a low-dose intermediate benzodiazepine such as lorazepam prn for agitation, as medication titration (any medication) is underway.
- Augment a mood stabilizer with a novel antipsychotic (i.e., a different class of medication with a bipolar designation).

Monitoring

It is prudent to formally check for change in target symptoms at each visit. During dose titration, it may be best to schedule weekly visits for the first month, even for med checks. A medication check [Clinical Procedural Terminology (CPT) 90862] also involves asking about any self-observed changes in health, obtaining blood pressure and pulse, and inquiring about any changes or additions of medications, including over-the-counter medications. A rough guideline for a 15-minute medication check, based on clinical trial experience, is to spend about a quarter of the time discussing interim life changes and stresses, half of the time reviewing symptoms, possible adverse effects, and relevant examinations, and the last quarter of time explaining changes or providing further psychoeducation.

For antipsychotics it is prudent to review health and changes in life situations at least annually, and periodically obtain weight, blood pressure, pulse, and metabolic syndrome parameters. Blood pressure (BP) monitoring should include at least one orthostatic blood pressure reading. Unlike some recommendations that suggest a 1- or 2-minute orthostatic reading, it is actually best to record the BP and pulse supine and immediately upon standing. If the BP falls, it should be recorded every 30 seconds until it either returns to baseline or until 2 minutes have elapsed. This measurement provides a general guideline regarding the period of risk if there is mild orthostatic change and determines whether the medication must be removed. Table 2.9 summarizes the areas and frequency of monitoring, as recommended by the American Dietary Association, American Psychiatric Association, American Association of Clinical Endocrinologists, and the North American Association for the Study of Obesity (2004).

Table 2.9. ADA/APA Monitoring Recommendations
for Antipsychotics

	Personal / Family History	Weight (BMI) (not required in guidelines)	Waist (in inches)	Blood Pressure	Hepatic Panel (not required in guidelines)	FBS and Fasting Lipid Profile
Baseline	X	X	X	X	X	X
1 month	X	X	—	X	—	—
2 months	—	X	—	—	—	—
3 months	—	X	—	X	X	X
Quarterly	—	X	—	—	—	—
Annually	X	—	X	X	X	—
Every 5 yrs	—	—	—	—	—	X

Note. ADA = American Dietary Association; APA = American Psychiatric Association; BMI = Basal Metabolic Index; FBS = Fasting Blood Sugar.

Additionally, hepatic enzymes should be followed periodically, usually after 3 months and then annually. A baseline EKG is also advisable to determine a baseline QTc and possibly avoid prescribing if the value greatly exceeds 450 msec (the cutoff used in most studies). Repeating the EKG depends upon the clinical situation.

Although there are no accepted guidelines for monitoring antidepressants, I follow the monitoring recommendations listed in Table 2.10, and obtain at least one orthostatic blood pressure check about 2 hours after every dose increase. An algorithm for which antidepressant medication should be considered first, and how to address later medication change decisions based on the NIMH sponsored STAR-D (Sequenced Treatment Alternatives to Relieve Depression) trial, is presented in Chapter 5. Generally, an annual metabolic panel is useful. The frequency of EKGs depends upon the patient's physical problems. An annual EKG would be useful only if there are relevant cardiac problems, such as the use of tricyclics that, because they are quinidine-like medications, may lead to heart blockage. Many antidepressants cause changes in blood pressure, so this should be monitored. It is adequate to substitute copies of the patient's routine medical labs and BP recordings as evidence of regular monitoring.

Table 2.10. Monitoring Recommendations for Antidepressants

	Personal / Family History	Weight (BMI)	Waist (in inches)	Blood Pressure	Hepatic Panel	EKG
Baseline	X	X	—	X	X	X
1 month	—	—	—	—	—	—
2 months	—	—	—	—	—	—
3 months	—	X	—	X	—	—
Quarterly	—	—	—	—	—	—
Annually	X	X	—	X	X	—
Every 5 yrs	—	X	—	X	—	X

Note. BMI = Basal Metabolic Index; EKG = Electrocardiogram Graph.

Mood stabilizers require similar periodic safety checks, as noted in Table 2.11, in addition to blood level screening. Screening blood levels for lithium or anticonvulsants is useful in preventing levels associated with potential side effects. A complete metabolic panel (CMP) and complete blood count (CBC) are needed because of the high rates of blood dyscrasias or hepatic side effects from many mood stabilizers.

Table 2.11. Monitoring Recommendations for
Anticonvulsant Mood Stabilizers and Lithium

	Personal / Family History	Weight (BMI)	Waist (in inches)	Blood Pressure	CMP and CBC	Blood Levels
Baseline	X	X	X	X	X	X
1 month	—	—	—	—	—	X
2 months	—	—	—	—	—	—
3 months	—	—	—	—	—	X
Quarterly	—	—	—	—	—	—
Annually	X	X	X	X	X	X
Every 5 yrs	—	—	—	—	—	—

Note. BMI = Basal Metabolic Index; CMP = complete metabolic panel (hepatic screen, BUN, creatinine, protein, blood sugar); CBC = complete blood count. Blood levels are specific for the medication; aim for therapeutic windows used for seizure medications.

Agitation

For elderly patients who are agitated, calming without sedation (sleep) is the goal, except for severe aggression. High doses of sedatives can obtund patients for hours to days. A model for calming without sedation was recently approved by the FDA for aripiprazole agitation in schizophrenia and bipolar mania (Andrenzina et al., 2006; Tran-Johnson et al., 2007) and is presented here because it is the same model recommended for agitation in geriatric patients (although doses and efficacy cannot be assumed to be the same). This methodology reflects best practice.

- Choose the same medication that you plan to continue. View the initial phase as "loading" or rapid dose titration. Do not use haloperidol, because of a higher side effect profile.
- Monitor target symptoms (not just global change). For example, agitation was defined two ways in the schizophrenia and bipolar mania trials. The primary outcome measure was the PANSS-EC (Positive and Negative Symptom Scale— Excitability; Kay, Fiszbein, & Opler, 1987), which contains the five items related to agitation: uncooperativeness, poor impulse control, hostility, excitement, and tension. The sec-

ondary measure was a global measure of agitation versus sedation (Meehan et al., 2001), which was a 9-point rating scale, from marked agitation to deep sleep to being unarousable.

- Consider the delivery system (form of medication). IM medications allow a consistent delivery system (100% of the medication is absorbed; none can be spit out), and have the most rapid onset of action (start within 30 minutes of the injection). IM also seems to have the strongest placebo effect (highest placebo response), and calming may occur with lower dosing.
- Administer the minimum effective dose used in studies.
- The IM dose could be repeated every 2 hours for up to two more injections or the maximum daily dose recommended for the medication. In virtually all studies of oral or IM treatments, initial change is seen within 30 minutes but does not really become statistically different from placebo until about 1 hour, with maximum effect by 2 hours. (Although not allowed in trials, clinical judgment should be used in practice if no initial change is seen within 30 minutes. This usually means the initial dose is too low and the repeat dose may be needed sooner than 2 hours.)
- Conversion to oral doses should be done as quickly as possible, although agitation due to delirium may not need continued treatment.
- IM or po lorazepam could be used if somnolence is desired for patient safety.

What is not known and requires further study is (1) IM to po conversion—that is, dose equivalents—when switching to maintenance, (2) duration of effects, and (3) the neurobiological basis of agitation to know, with certainty, which neurotransmitter systems or brain locations to target. Current choices are based on clinical judgment and extrapolation from other studies (off-label use).

SUMMARY

It is important to remember that geriatric psychopharmacology guidelines are based on existing studies and tests performed under optimal conditions. In practice, optimal conditions are rarely seen, thus, dose adjustments are based on knowledge of pharmacokinetic and pharmacodynamic changes with age. Sequential, single medication trials are the norm, although augmentation can be used cautiously. Benzodiazepines are not used as frequently due to adverse effects. Monitoring must be performed often and in more detail in elderly patients due to high rates of adverse effects. In the absence of specific clinical information, receptor affinity tables can help predict adverse effects and guide dosing changes. Psychoeducation is also crucial to improving compliance and reducing the fear that many older patients have of medication. These principles should be applied to all pharmacologic treatments described in subsequent chapters that deal with common psychiatric syndromes seen in elderly.

3

COGNITIVE DISORDERS: DIFFERENTIAL DIAGNOSIS AND TREATMENT

Dementia is defined as permanent, multiple cognitive deficits that include memory impairment and are caused by a general medical or neurological condition (American Psychiatric Association, 1994). Although dementia is mainly characterized by cognitive impairment, it is also associated with noncognitive behavioral disturbances. The psychosocial causes of behavioral problems (stress, lack of comprehension, lack of adequate structure, interpersonal conflicts) are common to all dementia patients, but there are also pathophysiological mechanisms that increase the risk for psychosis, depression, labile mood, violence, and impulsivity. Symptoms differ according to where the lesion occurs and often require treatment with psychiatric medications. Because of the similarities in treatment for behavioral disorders associated with all dementias, their cause and treatment are covered in Chapter 4 on the diagnosis and management of psychiatric symptoms associated with dementia and delirium. This chapter examines the differential diagnosis and treatment of cognitive disorders in late life.

OVERVIEW OF THE DEMENTIAS

An accurate diagnosis is required for cognitive impairment because the pathophysiology and hence treatment of cognition will differ in the future, even if they do not differ much now. Each dementia is characterized by the location where the main neuronal loss occurs. Cognitive symptoms are more pronounced in some dementias, whereas motor and sensory abnormalities dominate in others, and autonomic dysfunction in still others. Each dementia has a different neuropathology (i.e., pathological proteins, microscopic changes, and localization) and characteristic course of decline (rapid or slow, acute or insidious onset). The common dementias of late life are Alzheimer's, Parkinson's, Lewy body, vascular, and frontotemporal. Many less common disease states may cause cognitive impairment but are not covered here because of the lower frequency of occurrence. A final category of cognitive impairment is comprised of reversible conditions that mimic Alzheimer's, such as pseudodementia (cognitive impairment associated with depression, also called the dementia of depression), cognitive impairment associated with schizophrenia (dementia praecox), chronic delirium (cognitive impairment associated with medications), and normal pressure hydrocephalus (NPH).

Effective medication treatment for cognitive impairment is still at a relatively early phase of development for all dementias, although Alzheimer's has received the most attention. In treating cognition, medications are aimed at improving cognitive performance or affecting the course (slowing decline), but medications are rarely able to do both. Memory training and milieu interventions (structure, predictability, optimal stimulation) further maintain or improve function, but have more nonspecific effects.

Normal Changes versus Preclinical Disease

It is irrefutable that there are changes in cognition associated with aging. There was a longstanding debate among cognitive aging researchers as to whether such changes were real or artifacts of low education, changes in sensory systems (hearing, vision), changes in speed of processing, or disease. Some cognitive functions seem immune to change in normal older adults, such as verbal IQ, so these individuals might do equally well, compared to younger adults, if information in studies on cognitive function were presented differently and subjects were given more time to respond. Without modifications in presentation, normal older adults tend to show a decline in memory and in other functions, although they remain within the normal range of scores.

Differentiating early dementia from normal aging has received increased research interest as medications are developed to try to arrest neurodegenerative disease before it becomes symptomatic. Older adults often complain that they misplace objects such as keys more than they used to, are becoming forgetful, must make lists when they did not need to before, cannot "multitask" as well, and have increasing difficulty with name recall (e.g., of people, movies, books). If tested on a standardized memory test, individuals with age-associated memory impairment (AAMI) will score 1 standard deviation (SD) below the mean established for young adults (Crook et al., 1986). In AAMI, test scores are still within the range of normal, but are usually lower than expected for the individual's level of education and past success. The pattern of errors on neuropsychological tests (what they get wrong) is not the same as a clear cut Alzheimer's patient. Functional imaging studies such as computerized electroencephalograph (CEEG), positron emission tomography (PET), or functional magnetic resonance imaging (fMRI) are not sensitive enough to show definitive differences between AAMI and early dementia (i.e., cannot identify individuals who will get worse and "convert to dementia"). Note that an MRI is more routine and provides a static image of the brain, whereas an fMRI or PET show areas of the brain that are most actively metabolizing radioactively labeled glucose. Therefore, an fMRI or PET are usually performed only when there is a question about diagnosis after a routine MRI.

When cognitive changes are more severe but have not yet reached the severity of a dementia (threshold for diagnosis), the disorder is called mild cognitive impairment (MCI). On a screening test such as the Mini-Mental State Examination (MMSE), MCI patients score above the cutoff for dementia (below 24 on the MMSE). About 20% of MCI patients per year may evolve to a dementia level, but in the end, 20% will never get worse, making it clear that MCI is not necessarily an early manifestation of dementia. What causes the difference between no impairment, MCI, and progression to dementia is not still clear.

Cognitive Tests

A formal cognitive assessment must be performed and documented during the first session of an evaluation for an older adult. Many short cognitive test instruments are available. Commonly used scales are, as mentioned, the MMSE and clock drawing, although these are not ideal because they do not meet many of the following criteria for a clinically useful office test:

- Standardization (widely applied and administered in a similar way everywhere).
- No ceiling or floor effect (a *ceiling effect* is a test that is so easy that a score of 100% does not rule out early dementia; a *floor effect* is a test that is so hard that a score of 0% occurs even in mild cases and cannot differentiate between mild and severe disease).
- Contains the main diagnostic elements for dementia, as defined in the DSM-IV, namely: "multiple cognitive deficits that include memory impairment and at least one of the following cognitive disturbances: aphasia, apraxia, agnosia, or a disturbance in executive functioning. The cognitive deficits must be sufficiently severe to cause impairment in occupational or social functioning and must represent a decline from a previously higher level of functioning" (American Psychiatric Association, 2000).
- Meaningful norms (either has cutoff scores or probabilistic levels given for abnormal responses)
- Relatively short to administer
- Has good face validity (patients don't think it is too hard, and they think the questions are reasonable to ask)

Genetic and Medical Tests

Genetic typing will probably provide a major way of classifying many dementias in the future. At the present time, genetic tests mainly improve our certainty of diagnosis when symptoms are already present. For example, homozygous Apo e_4/e_4 is associated with a fourfold higher risk of AD, but many people with Apo e_4/e_4 do not develop the disease. ApoE testing is helpful if a diagnosis of AD is uncertain, but it is not diagnostic of AD if there are no cognitive symptoms. A urine test for AD that measures AD7c-NTP (a neural thread protein that is elevated in AD) has been marketed for many years, but involves the same constraints as ApoE testing. Generally, if genetic testing is felt to be necessary, such as ApoE subtyping, it is probably best to refer to a memory disorders program. Increased genetic knowledge and understanding of how each gene acts will ultimately lead to more specific treatments, if not a cure, for AD. Analogous findings are true for other common chronic dementias.

Medical and neurological evaluations are usually performed before the patient is referred to psychiatry. However, it is the responsibility of the psychiatrist to assure that an adequate medical/neurological workup has been performed (i.e., get a copy of the reports). Referral to neurology or other specialties is highly recommended if abnormal neurological findings or tests are discovered. As noted, laboratory tests such as genetic testing presently help most in confirming a diagnosis, but are not specific enough to be diagnostic by themselves.

Functional imaging (PET, CEEG, fMRI) improves the ability to make an early diagnosis but shows relatively low sensitivity (i.e., may be normal in early disease) or low specificity (i.e., may be abnormal in many conditions). Like other tests, imaging is useful in conjunction with abnormal neuropsychological testing for early diagnosis.

Differential Diagnosis of Dementia

The diagnosis of dementia is still based on clinical symptoms. As related above, it is not made because of an abnormal laboratory test or MRI. If a patient has significant cortical atrophy on an MRI, it would not be diagnosed as AD unless there were clinical symptoms. There are diagnostic criteria for each disorder that involve the presence of key symptoms and a typical course, and may be supported by specific tests such as neuropsychological testing patterns, imaging, or genetic testing in the near future. Imaging is the most important confirmatory test at the present time because the areas of the brain affected by the disease can largely explain the types of symptoms that will be manifested in a dementia.

Although "cognition" involves the integration of many brain areas—sensory input, information processing, and motor responses—presumed control centers are the hub for different cognitive functions. Subtypes of memory, for example, such as explicit memory (conscious) versus implicit memory (procedural and unconscious), have been assigned to certain brain centers (see Table 3.1) although it is really more complex.

Table 3.1. Neuroanatomy of Memory

Medial temporal lobe (diencephalons)	Explicit declarative memory (facts and events, textbook learning and knowledge)
Striatum	Procedural memory (skills and habits—e.g., automatically dialing a phone number but being unable to recite it)
Neocortex	Implicit memory (recall if primed or reminded by cues)
Amygdala	Emotional responses (involved in classical conditioning—pairing a stimulus with an emotional response and behavior)
Cerebellum	Skeletal musculature memory (involved in classical conditioning—pairing a stimulus with an emotional response and behavior)
Reflex pathways	Nonassociative learning (e.g., developed skill in a sport or musical instrument)
Parietal (Wernicke's area)	Speech comprehension (receptive)
Temporal (Broca's area)	Speech production (expressive)
Occipital cortex	Visuospatial integration

Source: From Zola-Morgan & Squire (1993).

Tables 3.2 and 3.3 show differences in clinical presentation between the different, common dementias. In general, the different diseases can be differentiated by the following presentation:

- Alzheimer's—insidious onset, gradual decline, recent memory is worse than remote memory; the memory disturbance occurs before incontinence, which precedes ataxia.
- Normal pressure hydrocephalus—gait disturbance occurs before incontinence, which precedes the dementia, and the progression is rapid.
- Vascular dementia—abrupt onset, stepwise deterioration, variable symptoms.
- Lewy body dementia—triad of memory disturbance, Parkinsonism (usually rigidity), and visual hallucinations is the most frequent pattern; decline is rapid (3 times the rate of AD).

Table 3.2. Patterns of Dysfunction in Chronic Dementias

	ALZHEIMER'S DEMENTIA (AD)	PARKINSON'S DEMENTIA (PD)
Executive functions	Impaired late (worse as the disease progresses)	Slow, set-shifting*
Memory	Recent > remote impairment; poor recognition recall	Slow processing speed; memory improved by cues (recognition recall)
Orientation	Disorientation to time precedes disorientation to place, and last to person	Variable (often global)
Language	Decreased fluency and word finding	Hypophonia (soft voice), micrographia, slow speech
Visuospatial function	Typically impaired early	Usually intact early
Motor	Intact early	Bradykinesia, rigidity, tremors early
Behavior	Apathy common, variable agitation, psychosis and depression (~ 30%)	Depression (~ 50% prevalence rate)
Onset	Insidious	Insidious
Course	Slowly progressive; cognitive impairment first; incontinence later; gait disturbance last	Slowly progressive
Comment	Possibly 3 MMSE points per year decline; usually tries to hide deficits	

* Set-shifting is the capacity to change attention from one task to another; the opposite is only being able to perform one task at a time. This capacity can be tested in a connect-the-dot (trail-making) task of connecting dot 1 to dot A, A to 2, 2 to B, B to 3, 3 to C, and so on. Many other methods exist to test this ability to switch between two sets of information quickly.

Table 3.2. (continued)

LEWY BODY DEMENTIA	MULTI-INFARCT DEMENTIA	FRONTOTEMPORAL DEMENTIA
Impaired early	Variable impairments	Decreased judgment and initiation early
Poor, similar to AD	Variable impairments	Intact early
Disorientation to time precedes disorientation to place, and last to person	Variable (sometimes no disorientation)	Intact early
Decreased fluency and word finding	Intact early	Decreased fluency, stereotypic speech
Copying good; drawing from memory poor	May be intact	Intact overall; poor planning ability
Rigidity and bradykinesia, less tremor (all more mild than PD)	Intact early	Intact early ("frontal gait" later)
Psychosis; usually prominent visual hallucinations	Often mild depression	Personality disturbance; impulsive and socially inappropriate
Insidious	Acute	Insidious
Rapidly progressive MMSE, possibly 10 points per year	Stepwise decline Hachinski scale is the common clinical scale	Slowly progressive
Mixed features of PD and AD		Behavioral disturbances are most prominent—"dirty dementia"—i.e., executive function deficits and self-neglect precede cognitive impairment

Source: Adapted from unpublished handout by John Mendoza (2005).

- Parkinson's dementia—occurs late in the course and involves global cognitive impairment.
- Pseudodementia—abrupt onset associated with a negative life event; errors are usually due to omission (refuses to answer); cognition improves as the interview progresses.
- Schizophrenia—cognitive dysfunction pattern is similar to AD, but there is no cortical atrophy, and symptoms may wax and wane.
- Chronic delirium—defined as chronic mild-to-moderate cognitive impairment due to sedative medications; concentration and new learning are especially impaired; ataxia and falls may occur; there is no improvement until removal of the offending agent.

Table 3.3. Patterns of Dysfunction in Potentially Reversible Conditions

	PSEUDODEMENTIA (DEPRESSION)	DEMENTIA OF SCHIZOPHRENIA
Executive functions	Minimal impairment	Severe impairment
Memory	Global impairment	Recent > remote memory impairment
Language	Decreased fluency (mutism)	Often echolalia, paucity
Visuospatial function	None	Often present
Motor	Psychomotor retardation	No impairment
Behavior	Anergy, apathy, often anxiety	Variable due to psychosis
Onset	Acute	Insidious
Course	Variable course	Gradual decline
Comment	Errors of omission rather than commission (refuse to answer or "I don't know" rather than true errors); they point out their errors (unlike AD); disorientation to both time and place seen early	No atrophy on MRI

Source: Adapted from unpublished handout by John Mendoza (2005).

Diagnostic Process

Unlike a traditional psychiatric interview that would focus on the patient's perception of problems (e.g., chief complaint, history of present illness, social history, stresses), the dementia assessment primarily focuses on mapping deficits, social skills, coexisting medical problems, and course without making the patient feel assaulted or stupid. It is also necessary to probe for psychiatric symptoms because affective disturbance, psychosis, and aggression are much more common in all dementias. Observations from caregivers are helpful, and degree of caregiver stress as well as the family's ability to provide appropriate care must also be assessed.

Table 3.3. (continued)

CHRONIC DELIRIUM	NORMAL PRESSURE HYDROCEPHALUS
Severe early impairment	Impaired early
Global impairment	Impaired late
Slurred or no impairment	No impairment
Not characteristic	Impaired late
Falls or no impairment	Impaired early (gait)
Variable—often depression	Variable—anergy, depressive symptoms
Acute (onset of meds)	Insidious
Stable	Slow progression (months)
Defined as being due to sedatives; concentration and registration of information are most impaired; no change until offending agent is removed	Usual progression is gait and neurological impairment first, incontinence second, dementia late; slow progression in motoric signs, no clear pattern for cognitive decline

The goal of the assessment is to confirm the most likely cause of the cognitive disturbance, the level of supervision and help needed, and how to best address behavioral symptoms and caregiver distress.

To allow maximum use of time in the first session for the interview and formal assessments, it is useful to have patients or families complete previsit information. The use of standardized tests improves the reliability of findings, but it must be remembered that the "gold standard" for all tests is still the skilled clinician.

Previsit Questionnaires
As noted, it is helpful to have patients/families fill out forms on the course of symptoms, health, function, doctors' contact information, and medications before the first session. These are pieces of information that few families remember without looking up. An introductory letter with the appointment date, map to the office, and instructions on how to complete the forms should be sent before the initial evaluation. The instructions should ask the patient to fill out as much as he or she can as part of the functional evaluation, and inform family members that they can correct or add to the information after the patient has finished. This process is actually part of evaluating the patient's baseline function. This preparatory work has the secondary benefit of reducing the patient's anxiety and involving him or her in the assessment early. Patients can bring the forms with them rather than sending them in before they arrive. Sample forms that I use are in Appendix 1 and can be used without permission (health screening—review of systems [ROS], list of current medications and doses, current and past psychiatric and dementia medications and adverse effects, list of doctors, a brief questionnaire on course and workups that have been performed).

First Visit
It is important to meet with the patient first and the family later, following the format used for the Clinician Interview Based Impression of Change—Plus (CIBIC-Plus), which is a semistructured interview format developed for AD clinical trials. If the patient insists on having one or more family members present, they should be instructed not to answer for the patient or help in any way. The family should still be seen alone at some point to clarify patient history and level of functioning.

Questions with AD patients should focus on the "here and now." Eliciting current symptoms such as pain or anxiety or gently confronting the patient about deficits he or she has just exhibited provides more meaningful information than global questions such as "Do you have any problems with your memory?" Observation of gait, tremor, asymmetry, neurological signs, mannerisms, and review of recent neurological and medical examinations should be made. A complete mental status examination, including thought process, mood, affect, receptive and expressive speech, content of speech, concentration, judgment, and insight, should be performed. Most importantly, a formal mental status examination, such as the MMSE, plus an executive function measure, such as the clock drawing task, should be conducted.

Gathering collateral information and evaluating family stress are the goal of family informant interviews. There are often discrepancies between family observations and the patient's self-report. However, because family accounts are not always totally accurate either, judgment must be exercised in determining the "real answer."

This type of evaluation often requires multiple visits or multidisciplinary evaluations. A memory assessment program should provide direct assessments (not just questionnaires), cognitive testing, family interviews, medical examination, and other evaluations. For example, in a memory assessment program, a social worker evaluates the family, a psychiatrist assesses the patient, a psychologist performs testing, an occupational therapist performs a direct functional assessment, and physicians from neurology and medicine may be involved if referral information is not complete. Additional imaging and testing can be ordered, if needed. This type of multidisciplinary assessment is difficult but not impossible to obtain in a solo office setting. Referrals for such measures are usually made when the initial office evaluation has left residual doubt about diagnosis, a clinical trial is desired, or psychoeducation or psychiatric treatment is anticipated.

Patient Fears and Potential Legal Issues

Many older adults are terrified of a dementia diagnosis and usually feel there is a lot at stake in receiving such a diagnosis. They are afraid of embarrassing themselves ("I hope I never get like that"), losing control of their finances and decision making, and being forced into a nursing home. Performance anxiety can make scores much worse. A school-like test situation is especially daunting for older adults with limited education. If guardianship is granted, patients lose their civil rights. For this reason, it is important to spend extra time explaining what will take place in the session, the purpose (that there are now treatments to improve memory), and trying to put the patient at ease for maximal performance. The use of naturalistic observations from the interview should be a part of the evaluation.

If the assessment is primarily for the purpose of determining competency or guardianship, the patient must still agree to share the information—unless the assessment is ordered by a court. The psychiatrist represents the patient, unless ordered by a court. In one instance in which a patient was contesting guardianship, an Advocacy Center lawyer was assigned who had the court disallow any hospital records or testimony from the treating doctors unless they were appointed by the court to regather the information. The information was collected again, but the process required considerable delays.

A common reason for an evaluation of early dementia is the experience of work-related difficulties due to memory problems, or behavioral problems associated with memory problems. Another common reason is the experience of getting lost going to familiar places. Guardianship is usually sought to protect a patient's financial assets, but family desire to control assets may not be altruistic. Sharing information with family without the patient's permission in any of these circumstances violates Health Insurance Portability and Accountability Act (HIPAA) regulations. Implicit consent can be proven if the patient approves the family meeting and is present at the meeting when giving information or planning treatment. This circumstance guards against later accusations of violating the patient's privacy or worse, abetting potential financial victimization.

CASE EXAMPLE

Mrs. A was an 83-year-old wealthy widow whose daughter was seeking guardianship. The daughter claimed that she needed to protect her mother's assets because of her dementia. Mrs. A was not only a wealthy woman, but she had started dating a man in his 70s and talked openly about intimate details with her daughter. The daughter was horrified by her mother's inappropriate behavior.

The patient had been seeing a general psychiatrist for depression and anxiety, and she was started on donepezil after complaining about cognitive impairment during her depressive episode. No formal mental status examination or neurological examination was recorded. The patient was still handling her own financial affairs, had a trusted investment advisor, was driving without an accident or getting lost, and still held active leadership positions in community organizations. She contested guardianship. In formal evaluations for her defense, after stopping donepezil for over 6 months, she scored 29 on an MMSE and in the normal range on a series of cognitive tests administered by a neurophysiologist. An MRI showed "changes normal for age" (minimal atrophy). Information was reported to the patient's designee (her lawyer) and the court, not the daughter or her lawyer directly. The patient had been labeled with AD because she had been given donepezil, and this alone was the main justification for the daughter's attempt to gain control of the mother's sizable assets. The case was dismissed.

ALZHEIMER'S DISEASE

Background

The diagnostic criteria for probable AD from the National Institute of Neurological Communicative Disorders and Stroke—Alzheimer Disease and Related Disorders Association (NINCDS-ADRDA; McKhann et al., 1984) are:

- Dementia (the loss of intellectual capacity and personality integration due neuronal loss)
- Established by clinical exam
- Documented by MMSE or similar examination
- Confirmed by other neuropsychological tests

- Deficits in two or more areas of cognition
- Progressive loss of memory and cognitive functions (e.g., language, motor skills, perception)
- No disturbance of consciousness
- Age of onset between 40 and 90
- Absence of systemic disorders or other brain diseases that could account for the deficits
- Supported by impaired activities of daily living (ADLs) and altered behavior patterns
- Supported by family history of similar disorders
- Supported by laboratory results (progressive atrophy on computerized tomography [CT] or MRI, normal LP, normal or nonspecific slowing on EEG)

Progression follows a consistent pattern and time course when not modified by medications or other concomitant diseases. One unique clinical staging measure was developed by Reisberg (1986) around functional deficits rather than cognitive deficits. The usual unmodified course from diagnosis until death is thought to be about 12 years, as noted in Reisberg's (1984) Functional Assessment Staging Test (FAST) of Alzheimer's Disease in Table 3.4.

Table 3.4. Functional Assessment Staging Test (FAST)

FAST STAGE	CHARACTERISTICS	APPROXIMATE DURATION	TYPICAL MMSE SCORE
1	No objective findings—subjective changes only (evolving preclinical changes)	50 years	30
2	Forgets location of objects, subjective work difficulties	15 years	30
3	Decreased functioning in demanding settings; difficulty traveling to unfamiliar locations	7 years	27
4	Cannot plan complex tasks (e.g., shopping)	2 years	24
5	Cannot select clothing; may require coaxing to bathe	18 months	18
6a	Difficulty dressing (e.g., buttons in wrong hole)	5 months	15
6b	Needs assistance bathing (fear of bathing)	5 months	13

Table 3.4 (continued)

6c	Difficulty with mechanics of toileting (e.g., may not wipe)	5 months	12
6d	Urinary incontinence	4 months	10
6e	Fecal incontinence	10 months	5
7a	Vocabulary limited to a few words	30 months	0
7b	Speech limited to a single, intelligible word	varies	0
7c	No intelligible vocabulary	12 months	0
7d	Needs support to sit	12 months	0
7e	Unable to smile	18 months	0
7f	Unable to hold head upright	Death	

Source: Adapted from Reisberg et al. (1984). Diagnosis of AD is usually made at stage 4.

Neurobiological Explanation

An explosion of research on AD now explains the gross and microscopic anatomical changes seen in the disease: namely, extracellular β-amyloid plaques and intracellular neurofibrillary tangles involving cholinergic cortical neurons in the parietotemporal area (greatest change) and, to a lesser extent, frontal and occipital lobes. Generally, it is assumed that memory and speech impairments are due to lesions in the parietotemporal areas; visuospatial impairments, to changes in the occipital lobes; and behavioral impairments, to frontal lobe changes.

β-amyloid is formed from an amyloid precursor protein (APP), which is a transmembrane protein present in neurons from birth (coded on chromosome 21). Amyloid plaques are dense precipitates of the β-terminal fragments (normally 40 amino acids long) when APP is broken down. β-amyloid in AD plaques consists of longer protein fragments than the normal soluble form (42–43 amino acids long). The plaques are surrounded by swollen neurons that contain microscopic tangles. The tangles are actually formed by the cross-linkages of abnormal hyperphosphorylated tau protein (tau protein usually stabilizes the microtubule assembly). Late in the course, β-amyloid is seen in the intimal layer of arteries (amyloid angiopathy), adding a vascular component to the disorder.

Many genetic abnormalities associated with AD involve coding abnormal APP sequences, or causing excess production of APP (chromosome 21), or cleaving APP in the "wrong place" (e.g., chromosome 14—presinilin 1; chromosome 1—presenilin 2), or facilitating cellular damage (e.g., ApoE, sortilin-related receptor, low density lipoprotein receptor class [SORL 1]) by increasing oxidative stress or intracellular calcium, or by facilitating apoptosis (cell death). Figure 3.1 shows the general sequence of changes in AD. The genetic abnormalities are becoming important in defining new medication treatment targets (Hardy, 2006; Hardy & Selkoe, 2002; Lukiw et al., 2000, 2005; OMIM, 2006; Rogaeva et al., 2007).

Figure 3.1. Amyloid precursor protein is cleaved by α, β, and γ secretases into β-amyloid fragments of 40–43 amino acid lengths, depending upon the APP sequences, isomorphic enzyme variation, and C-terminal fragments. APP = amyloid precursor protein; SORL 1 = sortilin-related receptor, low density lipoprotein receptor class.

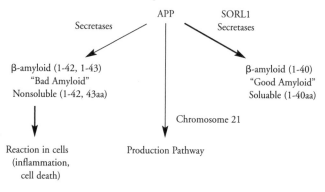

Normal versus Abnormal Behavior

The following neurological symptoms are *normal* in AD:
- Alexia (unable to grasp meaning of written material; also called visual aphasia)
- Aphasia (disturbance of language due to a brain lesion)
- Jargon aphasia (use of nonsense syllables or phrases)
- Agraphia (inability to communicate in writing)

- Mutisim (inability or voluntary refusal to speak; the counterpart of agraphia)
- Acalculia (inability to perform arithmetic operations; a parietal lobe retrolandic lesion)
- Agnosia (parital or total inability to recognize objects or how to use them)
- Anomia (inability to name objects or recognize spoken names of objects)
- Stereotypical speech (fixed, unvarying form of speech; use of the same phrase for every answer)
- Logorrhea (pathologically incoherent, repetitious speech or incessant, compulsive talkativeness)
- Confabulation (gives false stories to fill gaps in memory and feels the stories are true)
- Ecolalia (uncontrollable and immediate repetition of words spoken by another)

Other behavioral disturbances are always *abnormal.* The frequency of behavioral disturbances and depression is extremely high in AD. Although behavioral problems tend to increase as the disease progresses, behavioral symptoms, including depression and psychosis, may precede the diagnosis of AD by 6–18 months (Jost & Grossberg, 1996). As with frontotemporal dementia, changes in the frontal lobe and subcortical areas may account for behavioral disturbances.

The following problems need to be addressed as well:

- The risk of delirium is markedly increased.
- Driving hazard increases.
- Family support is necessary.
- Coordination with the primary care provider is necessary.
- Advance care planning (planning for the future) should be addressed.

Assessment and Diagnosis

No neuropsychological test is diagnostic of AD by itself. The cutoff score for probable dementia on the MMSE is a score below 24, with errors of disorientation, delayed recall, and visuospatial dysfunction, but the diagnosis must also meet NINCDS-ADRDA or DSM-IV criteria for the disorder.

The Alzheimer's Disease Assessment Scale—Cognitive (ADAS-Cog; Rosen, 1994) is a longer, commonly used, standardized cognitive instrument used in almost all AD medication trials. The ADAS has subtests for both cognition and behavioral disturbance, but only the 11-item cognitive function portion is generally applied. A point is given for every wrong answer, which means a perfect score is zero, and no correct responses total 70. Zero on the ADAS-Cog corresponds to 30 on the MMSE, and 70 on the ADAS-Cog corresponds to 0 on the MMSE. In clinical trials, mild dementia corresponds to about 14 on the ADAS-Cog and 20 on the MMSE.

The ADAS-Cog contains:

- A Word-recall task (immediate memory-concentration)
- Commands (e.g., "Make a fist")
- Constructional praxis (e.g., copy designs)
- Ideational praxis (e.g., prepare and send a letter)
- Delayed word recall (memory of the initial word list)
- Naming (speech)
- Orientation
- Cued recall (show a list of words, then show a second with only some of the original words on it to see how many are misidentified)
- General comments on remembering test instructions, coherence, word finding, and comprehension, and distractibility

For illiterate patients or for patients with poor English competency, the ADAS-Cog and even the simpler MMSE may not be reliable. For such patients, frequently the only recourse is to utilize simpler tests used for bedside screening that are thought to be more "culture fair." One such test is the Mini-Cog (Borson, Scanlan, Brush, Vitaliano, & Dokmak, 2000), in which the patient is asked to memorize three words, followed by a clock drawing task, followed by recall of the initial three words. Probable dementia is thought to be present if there are errors in recall of one or two words on delayed recall plus an abnormal clock drawing. A borderline score is one or two errors on delayed recall with normal clock drawing. In patients with Down's syndrome who are suspected of developing AD, there is a preexisting low baseline score that makes the usual test scores impossible to interpret unless there has been serial testing using the same measure. If the Rivermead Behavioral Memory Test was used, for example, serial declines of possibly 10% or more per year over a few years would be a useful cognitive measure.

Medicare guidelines allow for the tests listed in Table 3.5 to confirm the NINCDS-ADRDA criteria (Medicare, 2006).

Table 3.5. Tests Allowed by Medicare to Confirm
NINCDS-ADRDA Criteria

LABS

   B12 and folate blood levels (deficiency may cause dementia)
   Homocystein blood level (high or borderline high homocysteinemia is an
      increased risk for CVA or AD)
   Thyroid panel (TSH, T4, Free T3) (hypothyroidism may cause dementia)
   ESR (marker of inflammatory, infectious, autoimmune, and hyperviscosity dis-
      orders
   CBC with differential (evaluate anemia, cancers, infection, platelet disorders)
   Fasting chemistry panel (evaluate metabolic encephalopathy, calcium or
      parathyroid disorders, renal disease, diabetes, hypoglycemia, malnutrition
      or paraproteinemias, hepatic disease, and atherosclerotic disease)
   Urinalysis (evaluate for UTI)

IMAGING

   MRI if MMSE score is > 20 or onset of symptoms < 3 years (recent) or func-
      tions well (early).
   Contrast necessary if concerned about demyelinative disease or other indica-
      tions.
   Coronal slices perpendicular to temporal lobes are best to determine hippocam-
      pal atropy.
   Fluid-attenuated inversion-recovery (FLAIR) diffusion-weighted, and T2-
      weighted axial images are most useful for detecting white matter disease
      due to chronic cerebral ischemia or multiple lacunar infarcts.
   CT if severe cognitive impairment or MRI not possible. Same considerations as
      for MRI
   PET or SPECT [single photon emission computerized tomography] if MRI or
      CT is normal and early stage disease is suspected, or diagnosis unclear

CERTAIN CIRCUMSTANCES

   Apolipoprotein E genotype blood test if AD is uncertain or need to know the
      risk of heart disease, stroke, or AD (E4/E4 alleles).
   Blood ANA titer if elevated ESR or anorexia, weight loss, fatigue, undiagnosed
      anemia, arthritis, or skin rash.

Blood HIV titer if multiple sexual partners, IV drug abuse, or from sub-Saharan Africa.

Blood RPR if multiple sexual partners or history of sexually transmitted infection

EKG for suspected heart disease

CXR for smokers, exposure to asbestos, suspected tuberculosis, COPD or history of lung disease.

Estradiol for women (8 a.m.) if not on estrogen replacement therapy (ERT) AND postmenopausal or posthysterectomy with oophorectomy.

Plasma testosterone for men (8 a.m.) if symptoms of impotence, headache, insomnia, fatigue and weakness, swollen leg veins, or on testosterone-reducing medications such as Lupron or Medroxyprogesterone for prostate cancer.

Cerebrospinal fluid (CSF) for tau or beta amyloid (if diagnosis of AD versus frontotemporal dementia [FTD] needs to be determined)

Source: From Medical Care Corporation (2006).

Treatment Methods

Medications

The first generation of treatments involves replacement therapy of acetylcholine (ACh), the second generation of treatments focuses on glutamate modulation, and the third generation of treatments, still in development, will involve specific treatments based on genetic subtyping of AD.

Initial attempts to increase production of ACh in the brain via precursors for it, such as lecithin (phosphatidyl choline), did not prove effective. The use of acetylcholinesterase inhibitors (AChEI) allowed the best response to prevent the breakdown of ACh and prolong ACh effects at the synapse. Relative characteristics of the existing cholinesterase inhibitors are given in Table 3.6 and partially explain differences in effectiveness, side effects, duration of action, and risk of overdose. The first marketed cholinesterase inhibitor was tacrine (Cognex). It is an organophosphate, which is an irreversible agent related to nerve gases in World War I and certain insecticides. It is relatively irreversible and had systemic side effects, such as nausea, and parasympathetic side effects; it also had hepatic toxicity, which ultimately led to its withdrawal.

Table 3.6. Cholinesterase Inhibitors

	DONEPEZIL (Pfizer)	RIVASTIGMINE (Novartis)	GALANTAMINE (Janssen)
Dose (mg/day)	5–10 po qd	1.5, 3, 4.5, 6 po bid	4, 8, 12 po bid
Elimination Half-life ($t_{1/2}$)	70 h	1.5 h	1.5 h
Selectivity	AChE BChE	AChE nAChR	AChE
Bioavailability	100%	90%	40%
Protein Binding	96%	18%	40%
Metabolism	CYP2D6 CYP3A3/4 Glucuronidation	Glucuronidation	CYP2D6 CYP3A4
Reversibility	"Reversible"	"Reversible"	"Reversible"

Note. AChE = acetylcholinesterase; BChE = butyrlcholinesterase; nAChR = nicotinic acetylcholine receptor; CYP = cytochrome P450 pathway. Source: Adapted from Taylor (2001).

Butrylcholinesterase (BChE) is mainly distributed in the gastrointestinal system and muscle but is also present in brain. In AD there appears to be a shift of less AChE activity and slightly increased BChE activity in the hippocampus and memory areas of the brain. Postsynaptic nicotinic receptors seem to modulate ACh, increasing the strength of postsynaptic action potentials. Some clinicians believe that broader action of AChE (BChE and nicotinic action) will be more effective, although there have not been enough head-to-head comparisons to confirm differences. Time-release formulations have eliminated the need for twice-a-day dosing for rivastigmine and galantamine. Nausea is reduced by using time-release preparations or taking AChEIs with food.

The general recommendation is to start an AChEI when the diagnosis of AD is confirmed. The same cognitive test used at baseline should be repeated every dose change (monthly initially) and then every 3–6 months when on a stable dose. The patient should be checked for nausea and weight change at each visit. If the patient continues to worsen and not just plateau in response, change to a different AChEI. In general, start the patient at the lowest dose, to be taken with meals to avoid nausea. Increase the dose every 4–6 weeks until reaching the maximum tolerated dose or recommended maximum dose, whichever comes first.

If a patient has moderate AD, the addition of memantine is often tried. Memantine (Forest) is the first uncompetitive NMDA receptor antagonist controlling the NMDA receptor-operated cation (Ca^{++}) channels. Memantine is currently approved as a single agent for moderate-to-severe AD. When used in combination with donepezil, response seems superior than when either used alone (Tariot et al., 2004).

Referral for an AD clinical trial should also be considered to access new medications. Targets for new AD medications lie in immunotherapy, inhibitors of the inflammatory process to β-amyloid (e.g., COX-2 inhibitors, NSAIDS), reducing oxidative stress (e.g., vitamin E or C), reducing cholesterol and obesity, other glutamate modifiers, and other neuroprotective mechanisms (Reynolds & Mintzer, 2005).

Nonpharmacological Interventions for Cognition

Memory training using "mental exercises" such as puzzles or memory mnemonics may be useful in early stages but is not particularly helpful with moderate-to-advanced AD. Memory training teaches the use of traditional memory aids or mnemonics. It involves repetition, writing things down in a notepad (not on free sheets of paper that are lost easily), keeping a calendar and clock in prominent places, having emergency phone numbers by the phone or clearly labeled on automatic dial, *not* using cell phones, which will be lost, and using bizarre associations, such as tying a string on a finger to remember something.

For more severe impairment, behavior modification techniques (conditioned learning) are still useful because procedural (implicit) memory appears to be comparatively intact even in more advanced states. This type of memory—the "how-to" memory of doing things that cannot be put into words, such as finding a place without knowing the address or street—is less affected by AD. Behavior modification involves providing positive reinforcement when the right behaviors occur, and ignoring the wrong behavior (*not* providing negative reinforcement). Conditioning may teach AD patients to remember to use their memory book, to use certain paths or find certain locations when lost (such as the dayroom), or a variety of other simple behavioral tasks. One technique used to train AD patients to remember to use external memory aids is called spaced retrieval (modified cueing) (Bourgeois et al., 2003). Extinguishing behaviors is harder and is usually accomplished by ignoring the negative behavior while reinforcing a substituted behavior through positive intermittent reinforcement (rewards). Because behavioral therapy is not intuitive to most people, development of such reinforcement paradigms usually requires a specialist.

Even daily activities are often points of frustration for AD patients. Although rarely discussed in this way, an old mentor, Robert L. Kahn, used to say that there are two principles to maximize cognition and function in AD:

• Assure minimal intervention.
• Provide failure-free activities.

Minimal intervention does not mean allowing patients to neglect personal hygiene (bathing and dressing) or eating, but to avoid (1) forcing a patient into a nursing home for supervision against his or her will, (2) getting into power struggles over activities and schedules, or (3) infantilizing a patient by doing everything for him or her. Autonomy should be maximized for as long as possible, and providing only the assistance that people need. AD patients usually will not ask for help, so providing the right amount of help comes from knowledge of patients' capacities and personalities.

Failure-free activities involve only tasks that patients can still do well. Care has to be taken to avoid activities that patients view as childish or mere busy work. Application of Montessori-based methods may be useful to provide patients with cognitive stimulation and a sense of success by meaningfully interacting with physical and social environments on a regular basis (Camp, 1999). The Montessori method was developed in the early 1900s to educate children with mental disabilities. It espoused the creation of a special environment with clean, bright, stimulating materials that children would want to explore, and followed a guided discovery approach that required careful planning and direction.

Montessori-type examples for patients with AD include playing blackout bingo to stimulate memory and enhance motor and socialization skills; arranging flowers, watering plants, polishing a mirror, or setting the table to enhance care of the environment; working with clay, helping to measure or sift flour during a group cooking task to enhance gross motor activities (squeezing, scooping, pouring); and sorting tasks such as toolbox sorting and picture sorting to enhance recognition and categorization abilities.

Table 3.7 summarizes the recommended guidelines for psychosocial care.

Table 3.7. Principles of Psychosocial Care for Patients with AD

BASIC TENETS
1. Minimize intervention (have patients do as much as they can for themselves and avoid services they don't want).
2. Maximize a sense of control (empower or enable).
3. Pay attention to nonverbal communication (often a change in behavior is a sign of physical illness or discomfort).
4. Strive to provide failure-free activities, but not so simple that they are infantilizing.
5. Maintain social involvement.

ENVIRONMENTAL CONDITIONS
1. Provide structure (expectability).
2. Provide optimal stimulation (agitation can occur if patients are bored or overstimulated).
3. Emphasize activity (e.g., if patients are chair bound, they should have something within reach that they like to manipulate or like to do).
4. Avoid physical restraints.
5. Avoid clutter.
6. Safety proof rooms as the patient becomes more impaired (no dangerous objects such as guns or knives within reach; disconnect the stove; lower water heater temperature; hide car keys, etc.).
7. Simplify the number of choices (usually two, not three or four choices).

EXAMPLES OF ACTIVITIES FOR ADVANCED DEMENTIA
1. Sensory stimulation (simple recreational activities)
2. Music, art, pets
3. Audiotapes/DVDs (nature shows, favorite old TV shows without violence, family movies)
4. Therapeutic touch (manicures, tucking into bed, etc.)
5. Walks
6. Chair exercises (playing pass with a balloon or beach ball)
7. Small group socialization (e.g., family visits, day care)

Table 3.7. (continued)

8. Reality orientation/reminiscence (e.g., reading the newspaper, talking about family, parents, etc.)

Remember to keep activities short to match attention spans, and have many scheduled breaks.

Source: Adapted from Cohen-Mansfield (2001).

Supportive services become more important as the disease progresses. Senior centers for people with early dementia, adult day care, and respite programs (to allow caregivers a break) are all becoming increasingly available. These programs must be licensed and ordinarily are required to have minimum programming, staff ratios, and a nurse to administer medications. Transportation is usually available at a fee. Even former shut-ins find programs preferable to being alone and unsupervised or enduring the interpersonal intensity and cost of 1 sitter. If an AD patient is initially resistant to participating in the program, it is often helpful to let the caregiver attend the first day as a program helper.

PARKINSONS DEMENTIA

Background

Parkinson's disease (PD) is a chronic progressive disease caused by loss of greater than 50% of dopaminergic neurons in the nigrostriatal area. Motor symptoms predominate with bradykinesia (slowing of movement) progressing to akinesia (loss of physical movement) and tremor. Secondary symptoms may include impaired sense of smell, vivid dreams, autonomic dysfunction, poor proprioception (awareness of body position), pain (probably secondary to dystonia and rigidity), seborrheic dermatitis, urinary incontinence, constipation and gastrointestinal dysmotility, sexual dysfunction, and weight loss. Twenty to forty percent of patients are thought to develop dementia in the later stages of the disorder.

Neurobiological Explanation

A presynaptic neuronal protein called α-synuclein, which is normally soluble, aggregates to form insoluble fibril aggregates, called Lewy bodies, which appear to be neurotoxic. Genetic point mutations have been identified (A53T, A30P, E46K) that code for α-synuclein, and triplication of the gene causes some cases of Parkinson's disease (Polymeropoulos et al., 1997).

The loss of dopaminergic cells, which modulate the cholinergic system as well, and cortical cell loss as the disease progresses lead to cognitive impairment in the later stages.

Normal versus Abnormal Behavior

The disease can be difficult to diagnose accurately. Only 75% of clinical diagnoses of PD are confirmed at autopsy (Gelb, Oliver, Gilman, 1999). Psychiatric symptoms include daytime somnolence, insomnia (all phases), depression, speech disturbance, psychomotor retardation, and impaired reasoning, which may be exacerbated by medication effects.

Psychiatric symptoms in PD are common, particularly depression, anxiety, and agitation. Hallucinations are usually thought to be related to the use of dopaminergic agonists but can occur independently before medications are used. Dementia related to PD has a late rather early presentation.

Assessment and Diagnosis

The Hoehn and Yahr staging system (1967) has largely been supplanted by the Unified Parkinson Disease Rating Scale in studies (National Parkinson Foundation, 2007), but is presented in Table 3.8 because it is less complicated and more readily applicable for non-neurologists.

Treatment Methods

The only medication currently approved by the FDA for mild to moderate dementia associated with PD is rivastigmine (Exelon), although it is assumed that other medications in this class of medications may be useful. Doses are similar to AD (see Table 3.6).

Table 3.8. Parkinson Disease Stages

STAGE	MOTOR SYMPTOMS	PSYCHIATRIC SYMPTOMS
1	Mild, one-sided; others note change in posture and facial expression; generally tremor	Depression common
2	Bilateral symptoms, minimal disability	Depression common
3	Significant slowing, early impairment of equilibrium, moderately severe generalized dysfunction	Depression common
4	Severe, limited walking, rigid with bradykinesia, unable to live alone	Psychosis may be observed; depression common
5	Cachectic stage, invalidism, cannot stand or walk	Psychosis common; depression common

Source: Adapted from Hoehn & Yahr (1967).

DEMENTIA WITH LEWY BODIES

Background

The National Institute of Neurological Disorders and Stroke (NINDS; 2007) describes dementia with Lewy bodies (DLB) as

one of the most common types of progressive dementia. The central feature of DLB is progressive cognitive decline, combined with three additional defining features: (1) pronounced "fluctuations" in alertness and attention, such as frequent drowsiness, lethargy, lengthy periods of time spent staring into space, or disorganized speech; (2) recurrent visual hallucinations; and (3) parkinsonian motor symptoms, such as rigidity and the loss of spontaneous movement. People may also suffer from depression. The symptoms of DLB are caused by the build-up of Lewy bodies—accumulated bits of α-synuclein protein—inside the nuclei of neurons in areas of the brain that control particular aspects of memory and motor control. . . .

The similarity of symptoms between DLB and Parkinson's disease, and between DLB and Alzheimer's disease, can often make it difficult for a doctor to make a definitive diagnosis. In addition, Lewy bodies are often also found in the brains of people with Parkinson's and Alzheimer's diseases. . . . Like Alzheimer's disease and Parkinson's disease, DLB is a neurodegenerative disorder that results in progressive intellectual and functional deterioration. There are no known therapies to stop or slow the progression of DLB. Average survival after the time of diagnosis is similar to that in Alzheimer's disease, about 8 years, with progressively increasing disability.

Neurobiological Explanation

Alpha-synuclein accumulates into Lewy bodies, as in PD, and causes multiple system atrophy. The disorders in which α-synuclein accumulates in different brain regions are collectively referred to as "synucleinopathies." Family histories of DLB are rare, and it is not clear how Lewy bodies cause the particular symptoms of DLB.

Normal versus Abnormal Behavior

The classic behavioral manifestations of the disorder involve a triad of symptoms—cognitive impairment similar to AD, visual hallucinations as the most common psychotic symptom, and parkinsonism (usually rigidity rather than tremor). DLB has a much more rapid rate of decline (often doubled) than AD.

Assessment and Diagnosis

No special diagnostic tests are available. The clinical diagnosis is made by the pattern of symptoms and progression. Autopsy confirmation is the definitive diagnosis.

Treatment Methods

There is no cure for DLB. Levodopa for Parkinson symptoms (rigidity and loss of spontaneous movement) may be required but is minimized to reduce worsening of psychotic symptoms. Traditional antipsychotics for psychosis are minimized to reduce worsening of Parkinson symptoms. AChEI, such as donepezil, galantamine, and rivastigmine, are the main medications for cognitive symptoms of DLB and may reduce psychiatric and motor symptoms. Atypical antipsychotics seem superior in treating hallucinations without worsening Parkinson symptoms, but should be used at the lowest possible dose (Ballard, Grace, & Homes, 1998).

Psychosocial interventions are nonspecific and follow recommendations covered in Chapter 4 on behavioral disturbances in dementia.

VASCULAR DEMENTIA

Background

Vascular dementia (VaD) is often listed in the differential diagnosis of dementia, but only multi-infarct dementia (MID), which involves occlusion of small peripheral vessels, is confused with AD because it also has an insidious onset and gradual decline.

MID is usually differentiated from AD by its course. Typically there is a stepwise deterioration (abrupt changes and plateaus) involving small lacunar infarcts in key areas mediating cognition. Because the strokes often miss motor, speech, and sensory areas, they go unrecognized as acute brain attacks and are often difficult to differentiate from AD.

Neurobiological Explanation

VaD may be caused by large or small blood vessel occlusion, depending upon the location and extent of the areas being supplied. It includes Binswanger's disease and subcortical leukoencephalopathy ("subcortical ischemia"), AD with cerebrovascular features (not called mixed dementia anymore), lacunar lesions (several small strokes), and larger strokes. On imaging, strokes in any of the areas listed in Table 3.9 are likely to support a diagnosis of VaD.

Table 3.9. Obligatory Locations for VaD
(any one of the below)

LARGE VESSEL STROKES IN THE FOLLOWING TERRITORIES:
Anterior cerebral artery
Posterior cerebral artery involving paramedian thalamic infarctions or inferior
    medial temporal lobe lesions
Association areas involving paratemporal, temporo-occipital, or angular
    gyrus
Watershed carotid arteries in superior frontal or parietal regions
Large vessel lesions of the dominant hemisphere
Bilateral large-vessel hemispheric strokes

SMALL VESSEL DISEASE (LOCALIZATION):
Multiple basal ganglia and white matter lacunae
Extensive periventricular white matter lesions
Bilateral thalamic lesions
Leukoencephalopathy involving at least a quarter of total white matter

Source: Adapted from Roman et al. (1993).

Normal versus Abnormal Behavior

Neurological deficits are dependent upon the location of the lesion. With multi-infarct dementia, which can be confused with AD because motor impairment may not be seen, cognitive impairments are usually more patchy than in AD, with certain neuropsychological functions being relatively spared and others worsened. For example, a patient with MID may have severe functional impairment with relatively mild cognitive impairment, or severe speech hesitancy and memory problems but be relatively well-oriented.

There is often more than one potential cause for dementia, and each dementia must be coded separately. AD with cerebrovascular disease is reserved for patients who meet clinical criteria for possible AD but also present clinical or brain imaging evidence of a VaD. These patients with imaging changes consistent with VaD have been excluded from AD studies, irrespective of the course. Vascular changes also cause depression, especially with lesions in subcortical and frontal areas (Alexopoulos et al., 1997).

Assessment and Diagnosis

Thrombotic strokes involving large vessels have a so-called watershed pattern of injury on MRI. The area of infarction looks like a piece of pie, smallest at the point of occlusion and fanning out to include the entire area that the blood vessel supplied. The corresponding damage involves functions supplied by the artery. The stroke may show motor and sensory symptoms when the right middle cerebral artery is involved at its origin, but small vessel occlusions lead to patchy and diffuse symptoms, often mainly cognitive.

The NINDS-AIREN criteria for vascular dementia (National Institute of Neurological Disorders and Stroke and Association Internationale pour la Recherché et l'Enseignement en Neurosciences; Roman et al., 1993) requires focal neurological signs, radiological evidence of cerebrovascular disease, a temporal relationship between dementia and onset of focal neurological signs (within 3 months), and usually stepwise deterioration. Lacunar infarcts in areas that are not associated with cognition are unlikely to cause dementia symptoms. MRI findings of subcortical ischemic change are extremely common (periventricular hyperintensity on T2 weighted images), but are only considered possible VaD when it is severe enough to extend to the basal ganglia.

The Hachinski scale categorizes the type of changes seen in VaD (Hachinski et al., 1975) by assessing 13 items. The more heavily associated symptoms are abrupt onset, fluctuating course, history of strokes, and focal neurological symptoms and signs. Other features that differentiate it from AD are stepwise deterioration, nocturnal confusion, preserved personality, depression, somatic complaints, emotional incontinence, hypertension, and other evidence of systemic atherosclerosis.

Treatment Methods

Decline is variable and often dependent upon whether risk factors for stroke have been corrected (hypertension, obesity, hyperlipidemia, diabetes, and smoking) and prophylactic anticoagulants started.

No FDA approved medications are available for VaD,

although several small-N AChEI studies have been reported to have benefit without undue safety and efficacy problems.

FRONTOTEMPORAL DEMENTIA

Background

Frontotemporal dementia (FTD) includes Pick's disease, primary progressive aphasia, and semantic dementia. Although these have different labels because speech disorders may predominate in some, the pathophysiology is similar. Corticobasal degeneration and progressive supranuclear palsy have similar findings and are often called the "Pick complex."

Quoting from the website of the National Institute of Neurological Disorders and Stroke (2007):

> As it is defined today, the symptoms of FTD fall into two clinical patterns that involve either (1) changes in behavior, or (2) problems with language. The first type features behavior that can be either impulsive (disinhibited) or bored and listless (apathetic) and includes inappropriate social behavior; lack of social tact; lack of empathy; distractability; loss of insight into the behaviors of oneself and others; an increased interest in sex; changes in food preferences; agitation or, conversely, blunted emotions; neglect of personal hygiene; repetitive or compulsive behavior; and decreased energy and motivation. The second type primarily features symptoms of language disturbance, including difficulty making or understanding speech, often in conjunction with the behavioral type's symptoms. Spatial skills and memory remain intact. There is a strong genetic component to the disease; FTD often runs in families.

The disease generally progresses rapidly; the course may be as short as 2 years from diagnosis until death.

Neurobiological Explanation

FTDs are often labeled tauopathies because they have filaments of tau inclusions in neurons and glial cells (oligodendroglial cells and astrocytes), limited to the frontal lobes. Ubiquitin inclusion bodies are also seen (ubiquitin is an ATP-dependent proteolytic system), and there are ubiquitin positive–tau negative frontotemporal cases identified to challenge the notion of FTD as exclusively a tauopathy. Genetic mutations have been identified in the gene encoding microtubule-associated protein tau (MAPT; on chromosome 17) and other families of genes on chromosome 17. Like AD, abnormalities in the presenilin-1 gene on chromosomes 14 and 3 have been described (Mathuranath, 2007; OMIM, 2007).

The pathological intracellular changes cause cellular dysfunction and ultimately lead to free radical damage and neuronal cell death.

Normal versus Abnormal Behavior

Patterns of neuropsychological changes that differentiate this dementia from AD are disproportionately higher severity in social and executive dysfunction (decision making, appropriateness) compared to the level of cognitive dysfunction in declarative memory, working memory, visuoconstruction, processing speed, and semantic functions (Libon et al., 2007). There are still cognitive impairments, just less severe than in AD for the level of function. The Reisberg's FAST scale would not apply.

Like other chronic dementias, FTDs occur most commonly in elderly people but may also occur as a "presenile dementia"—that is, at a slightly younger age. FTDs are often nicknamed the "sloppy dementias" to characterize their presentation as an executive function disorder.

Assessment and Diagnosis

The diagnosis for FTD is a clinical one. Lab tests and imagining are used to help differentiate it from other dementias (disproportionate frontal atrophy, executive dysfunction, no lab abnormalities). It is especially important to note behavioral risks and supervision needs. As with AD, genetic subtyping of FTD should have significance in the future.

Treatment Methods

No medication treatments have been shown to slow the progression of FTD. Cognitive symptoms are often treated by off-label use of AChEI at the same doses as for Alzheimer's dementia, although benefit has not yet been proven. Based on personal communication with Don Royal, M.D. (2007), an expert on executive dysfunction, behavioral problems may be ameliorated by off-label use of SSRIs, but this usage has not yet proven either.

PSEUDODEMENTIA
(DEMENTIA OF DEPRESSION)

Background

There has been a longstanding observation of cognitive slowing and dementia-like symptoms with major depression. In elderly people, cognitive impairment caused by depression is often diagnosed as a dementia and is not treated appropriately. Although the actual mechanism of cognitive impairment in depression is not known, pseudodementia is not merely a misdiagnosis of indifference, apathy, and psychomotor retardation from depression. In pseudodementia, the affective component does not appear to be as severe as the cognitive deficits.

Neurobiological Explanation

The neurobiological causes of cognitive impairment in depression are probably related to dysfunction in serotonin, dopamine, and acetylcholine systems that form interconnected pathways between the frontotemporal cortex and subcortical areas and affect memory and behavior. There is also longstanding knowledge of limbic–hypothalamic–pituitary–adrenal dysfunction in depression with a loss of diurnal variation in cortisol and presumably adrenocorticotropic hormone (ACTH) and corticotropin releasing factor (CRF) as well (Elgh et al., 2006; O'Brien et al., 2004). Unlike normal subjects, depressed patients failed to suppress cortisol production in the morning after being given 1 mg of dexamethasone the night before (Coppen et al., 1983). The persistently high-normal cortisol levels and loss of diurnal rhythm that characterize this condition are associated with a smaller volume on the left prefrontal cortex in patients with major depressive disorder and schizophrenia, which may account for executive dysfunction and memory loss in these conditions (Coryell et al., 2005), although a causal link (actual chain of events or mechanism) is difficult to prove. It is likely that ACTH and CRF, which modulate glutamate response, may have the main influence on cognitive dysfunction.

There is a much higher rate of conversion to dementia in elderly patients who show depressive pseudodementia compared to cognitively intact depressed patients (71.4% vs. 18.2%; Saez-Fonseca et al., 2006), suggesting that pseudodementia may actually be a cardinal sign for early dementia.

Normal versus Abnormal Behavior

Depressive pseudodementia usually has a combination of depressive symptoms and cognitive symptoms. A diagnosis cannot be made without mood complaints or their equivalent. For example, mood-related signs include ruminations, worries, persistent sad expression, tearfulness, lack of reactivity to pleasant events, and irritability. Neurovegetative signs include appetite loss, weight loss, lack of energy, cyclic patterns (diurnal variation), sleep disturbance, and early morning awakening. There may also be ideational disturbances with feelings that life is not worth living, self-depreciation, excess pessimism, or preoccupations with health. All of these symptoms may be reported even as the patient denies feeling depressed.

Cognitive problems seem different from those associated with AD. More errors of omission (won't answer), psychomotor retardation, and more variability and less disorganization in learning (semantic memory) are noted in pseudodementia, and these symptoms improve during the interview because of the interest shown (Wells, 1979). In some cases, there are complaints of excessive memory loss, but patients actually show no measurable memory deficits (Yousef et al., 1998).

Patients with pseudodementia usually have a history of depression, but the presentation is different from prior episodes. There is also usually a psychosocial stressor triggering the changes.

Unique Aspects of the Disorder in Elderly

Cognitive disruption associated with depression in younger people is usually related to the severity of the disorder. In elderly patients mood complaints may sometimes appear mild in comparison to the cognitive disturbance.

Assessment and Diagnosis

Although the dexamethasone suppression test (DST) was administered to improve diagnosis of atypical depression in the 1980s, it was found that the test produced abnormal levels in stress-related disorders as well as dementia and was therefore a fairly nonspecific finding.

The diagnosis is still a clinical one. The most recent pseudodementia scale, by Yousef et al. (1998), largely quantifies subjective differences in the history (recurrent depression, diurnal variation, avoidant personality style, sleep and appetite disturbance, relatively sudden onset and rapid decline), insight (poor), and quality of responses (variable patterns, poor concentration, errors or omission, improve as the interview progresses).

Treatment Methods

There is generally no difference from the usual treatment approaches for depression. Use of AD medications is not needed, unless it becomes clear after depression treatment that there is an underlying dementia.

DEMENTIA PRAECOX (COGNITIVE IMPAIRMENT ASSOCIATED WITH SCHIZOPHRENIA)

Background

The term *dementia praecox*, which is synonymous with the current term *schizophrenia*, was coined by Emil Kraepelin (1893) to describe a peculiar condition of mental weakness occurring at a youthful age.

Disorganized thinking, delusions, and hallucinations are hallmarks of schizophrenia and remain core features in the DSM-IV-TR.

Significant cognitive impairment and deterioration are observed in people with chronic schizophrenia as they age (Friedman et al., 1999; Morrison et al., 2006). Both cortical (language and memory) and subcortical (negative symptoms) disorders may appear very similar to AD symptoms, but there are no neuropathological changes of AD (no plaques or tangles or significant atrophy; Harvey et al., 2002).

Neurobiological Explanation

A variety of abnormalities in neurotransmission has been identified in schizophrenia that may account for cognitive impairment, including dopamine (D_1) receptors, norepinephrine (NE) and dopamine transporters, catechol-O-methyltransferase (COMT) genotype, and acetylcholine. White matter abnormalities and abnormalities in distribution of gray and white matter have also been predictive of patterns of memory impairment (Harvey, 2005). However, no standard lesions can be reported.

Normal versus Abnormal Behavior

A review by Friedman et al. (1999) described the following changes in older adults with schizophrenia:

- Global cognitive performance declines by an average of 3 MMSE points per decade.
- More severe negative symptoms (Friedman et al., 1999).
- Compared to AD, less impairment in naming.
- Similar changes compared to AD in early severe impairments in memory, new learning, and visuospatial tasks.
- Similar to AD in relative early sparing of recognition, fluency, and clock drawing.

Unique Aspects of the Disorder in Elderly

Elderly adults with schizophrenia seem more functionally impaired than patients with AD who have similar cognitive deficits on testing (more severe negative symptoms).

Assessment and Diagnosis

The evaluation for cognition in schizophrenia is the same as a standard dementia workup. Generally, imaging does not reveal significant atrophy, and neuropsychological test patterns do not reveal significant pattern differences from AD.

Treatment Methods

There are no FDA-approved medications for cognitive impairment in schizophrenia. The first-line strategy at the present time is to use atypical antipsychotics because they are associated with less global cognitive and memory impairment. Clozapine seems to improve motor functions better than other atypicals but causes more impairment in global cognitive functioning. Categories of medications that have theoretical value and case reports of efficacy include the following (Harvey & McClure, 2006):

- D1 receptor agonists (largely distributed in frontal areas)
- $\alpha 2$ receptor agonists such as clonidine
- $\alpha 1$ receptor agonists
- AChEIs (donepezil and galantamine studied)
- Serontonin system (5-HT1A receptor partial agonists, 5-HT2A receptor antagonists, 5-HT4 receptor partial agnonists, and 5-HT6 receptor antagonists) all improved cognition in animal models.
- Gamma-aminobutyric acid (GABA) and the glutamate α-amino-3-hydroxy-5-methyl-4-isoxazoleproprionic acid (AMPA) inhibitors (e.g., memantine)

Nonpharmacological cognitive remediation has shown some benefit for younger patients with schizophrenia, and there is no reason to think that it would be less effective in older patients. Cognitive enhancement therapy (CET) was developed and piloted in the mid-1990s by Gerald Hogarty and colleagues (2004). This approach teaches cognitive skills such as perspective taking and social-context appraisal from unrehearsed *in vivo* social interactions. CET combines progressive software training exercises in attention, memory, and problem solving with weekly social-cognitive group exercises. This cognitive–behavioral therapy (CBT) technique proved quite effective over a 2-year follow-up (Hogarty et al., 2004).

NORMAL PRESSURE HYDROCEPHALUS

Background

Normal pressure hydrocephalus (NPH) is the cause of about 1% of dementia cases. The symptom progression of NPH is opposite the pattern seen in AD. It usually begins with ataxia (unsteady gait) and progresses to urinary incontinence, and finally dementia (cognitive impairment) later in the course, whereas AD begins with dementia, progresses to urinary incontinence, and finally to ataxia and other motor abnormalities. The time course for NPH is more rapid than AD, going from mild to severe within a matter of 1–2 years rather than 6–7 years.

Neurobiological Explanation

NPH results from a blockage of the normal flow of CSF, which is produced by the choroid plexus, mainly in the lateral ventricles, and circulates through the interventricular foramina into the third ventricle, then through the cerebral aqueduct into the fourth ventricle before exiting through several foramina over the cerebral hemispheres and down the spinal cord. It is reabsorbed by the arachnoid granulations in the venous system. CSF is produced at a rate of 500 ml/day. The most common conditions that can cause obstruction of the normal flow, usually into the third ventricle, are head injury, stroke, meningitis, or a brain tumor, but at least 60% of the cases do not have a clear etiology. Dementia results from distortion of the periventricular system, which in turn distorts underlying structures and function (Dalvi, 2006).

Normal versus Abnormal Behavior

Initial symptoms of NPH are subtle. Generally gait disturbance (unsteadiness, weakness, falls, shuffling, frontal gait, and freezing) precedes appearance of incontinence (urinary incontinence, but can involve fecal incontinence later), which precedes the dementia (memory loss, speech problems [usually fluency], apathy, mood disturbance, and difficulties with reasoning and judgment).

Assessment and Diagnosis

The standard dementia workup should suggest a pattern that is different from AD. It is important to obtain an MRI early, which shows ventricular enlargement with the cortex pushed outward. Cisternography—which requires a lumbar puncture to measure CSF pressure by following the distribution and reabsorption of a radiopaque solution injected into the CSF—is rarely done anymore.

Treatment Methods

NPH is treated with ventriculoperitoneal shunting, provided it is diagnosed early enough for reversibility. Psychiatric symptoms such as depression are common and do not respond to antidepressant treatment or psychotherapy.

DELIRIUM

Background

Delirium is by far the most common psychiatric abnormality caused by medical illness. It is characterized by an acute-onset disturbance of consciousness (attention and arousal) and cognition (memory, disorientation, language). Less severe delirium, with mild-to-moderate memory loss and concentration difficulty due to medications, is more common in outpatient practice. Delirium is usually missed without direct mental status screening. The reason to identify delirium early is that cognitive impairment may persist if not corrected rapidly.

Delirium is caused by global brain dysfunction during an illness. Those at highest risk for delirium include the following:

- Elderly individuals
- Postcardiotomy patients
- Burn patients
- Patients with preexisting brain damage (dementia, CVA)
- Drug-dependent patients (withdrawal)
- Patients with AIDS
- Sleep-deprived individuals (may just be a prodromal sign)
- Sensory-deprived individuals

Delirium is defined by four major criteria (American Psychiatric Association, 2000):

- Disturbance of consciousness
- Change in cognition
- Changes that evolve over hours to days
- Evidence for a medical basis (abnormal labs, physical examination)

Chronic cognitive impairment due to medications can mimic AD and can be considered a "chronic delirium" because it emerges shortly after starting the causal sedative medication, waxes and wanes with peak plasma levels, and does not improve until the causal agent is removed. Delirium may lead to irreversible damage. Ninety-eight percent of elderly patients who developed a delirium during hospitalization still showed cognitive impairment at the time of discharge, and 31.1% still showed cognitive impairment at 6 months postdischarge (Levkoff, 1992).

Neurobiological Explanation

Because excitatory neurotransmitters are active during delirium (NMDA, glutamate) and do cause glutamatergic neurotoxicity in animal studies, Stahls (2000) coined the term "glutamate storm" to describe the cellular damage presumed to occur from a chronic agitated delirium. Verification of abnormal brain activity can be obtained by EEG, although it is rarely necessary.

A recent review article on the interrelationship between delirium and dementia demonstrated multiple pathophysiological mechanisms for delirium (Marcantonio et al., 2006). The many triggers for the pathological changes include relative cortisol excess from stress, glutamate and GABA dysfunction, dopamine activation, cytokine excess, serotonin dysfunction, and cholinergic dysfunction—all cause cognitive dysfunction. All of these systems interact as feedback mechanisms and serve as inhibitory or excitatory neurotransmitters to facilitate neuronal function.

Presumably, cholinergic hypoactivity in the cortex may account for cognitive and psychotic symptoms; dopmanergic hyperactivity in the mesolimbic system accounts for hallucinations; serotonergic hyperactivity accounts for aggression and mood disturbance; and glutamate neurotoxicity ("glutamate storm") accounts for agitation and ultimately neuronal cell death.

Alcohol and medications, usually benzodiazepines, are the most common causes of "chronic delirium." Reduced GABA activity and glutamate activation are likely in alcohol or benzodiazepine withdrawal, and GABA activation with chronic benzodiazepine use. Other medications may affect cholinergic, serotonergic, or dopamine function.

Normal versus Abnormal Behavior

Attention and new learning are usually disproportionately affected. These areas are tapped by serial calculations (e.g., serial 7s) or digit span testing (most people can recall seven to ten numbers, such as a phone number). Speech may be slurred, and arousal may be difficult at times and inconsistent. Sleep disturbance such as daytime drowsiness and nighttime insomnia, as well as variability of symptoms (waxing and waning), are common.

Older adults are the most vulnerable group for developing a delirium because of the high rates of polypharmacy, medical comorbidities, and dementia. In a prospective hospital study, patients from nursing homes who were sicker and more likely to have a preexisting dementia, had a 64% rate of emergent delirium during a hospitalization compared to 24% of community dwelling, age-matched elderly (Levkoff et al., 1991). Sleep deprivation is also associated with delirium, although it is not clear if it is a risk factor or a prodromal sign.

Assessment and Diagnosis

Assessment requires history of the temporal onset and course, cognitive evaluation, and medical evaluation. The evaluation requires a detailed mental status examination in addition to observations and information from nursing staff or informants. Cognitive status changes usually include poor concentration, impaired speech (e.g., slurred articulation, loose content), disorientation (usually global—time, place, and other people), altered perceptions (e.g., illusions, delusions, or hallucinations), constructional problems, dysnomia, and dysgraphia. Olfactory hallucinations ("something burning") and visual hallucinations ("picking at the air") appear to be common, as well as haptic hallucinations ("something is crawling on my body"). Cognitive status can usually be ascertained by routine questioning, and a brief formal measure such as the Mini-Cog can be applied at periodic intervals. (Borson et al., 2000). As noted previously, this test involves memorization and recall of three words separated by an interference task of drawing a clock.

The presence of any of the symptoms listed in Table 3.10 warrants intensive medial attention and treatment.

Table 3.10. Delirium Rating Scale

- Temporal onset of symptoms (abrupt change over 1–3 days)
- Perceptual disturbances
- Hallucinations
- Delusions
- Psychomotor behavior (agitation severe)
- Cognitive status (acute deficits)
- Physical disorder implicated
- Sleep–wake cycle disturbance (fluctuating)
- Lability of mood (especially disinhibition)
- Variability of symptoms (wax and wane)

Source: From Trepacz (1985).

All likely causes must also be aggressively sought and treated. An MRI is indicated when a stroke or mass is suspected, but is otherwise normal. EEG is helpful in showing an encephalopathy, but the patient may be too agitated for functional testing. A screening of cognition, mood, blood pressure, and gait (through observation) should be done whenever a new medication is started that is known to have some cognitive influence.

There is usually more than one possible etiology for delirium, and each illness has to be treated simultaneously as if it is the cause (Francis, 1990). The most common causes of delirium are captured in the mnemonic I WATCH DEATH, which every medical student is taught.

I   = Infection

W = Withdrawal
A = Acute metabolic
T = Toxins, drugs
C = CNS pathology
H = Hypoxia

D = Deficiencies
E = Endocrine
A = Acute vascular
T = Trauma
H = Heavy metals

The Confusion Assessment Method—Intensive Care Unit (CAM-ICU) is a special scale that was developed to tap vigilance (hyperalertness), lethargy, stupor, and coma in patients who are intubated or nonverbal (Ely et al., 2001). History of the symptoms, observational items, an auditory recognition task and similarities task for attention and reasoning are included in the scale. Even in medical situations, drugs that might cause a cognitive impairment must be considered, especially pain medications.

Treatment Methods

Medications
It is believed that rapid calming will decrease the glutamate neurotoxicity underlying the relatively high rate of permanent cognitive impairment from delirium and, more importantly, is needed for patient safety and comfort in the midst of a delirium. The definitive treatment is management of the cause for the delirium.

If there is more than one possible cause, as is typically the case, all must be treated simultaneously.

There are no specific treatments for the cognitive impairment, although treatment with selective AChEIs used for AD but may protect against neurotoxicity (based on animal studies; Takada et al., 2003). Medication treatment for the behavioral aspect of delirium is covered in Chapter 4.

Psychosocial Interventions

In order to minimize antipsychotic use, general nonpharmacological (behavioral) approaches are applied, as summarized in Table 3.11.

Table 3.11. General Nonpharmacological Approaches

Improve environment—quiet, soothing environment; quiet music; avoid TV (especially shows with violent themes and noise).

Reorient cues (clock, calendar, newspaper, read to the patient, discuss current events)—for example, "When your daughter visited last night, she told me . . .").

Provide frequent one-to-one support—in a hospital setting it is better to have the delirious patient closer to the nursing station than at the end of the hall.

Provide ample nutrition and hydration.

Sleep—allow sleep but try to maintain a diurnal rhythm (less daytime naps if the patient is awake at night).

Avoid restraints (patients fight them)—it is better to safety proof the environment and involve the patient in group activities.

CASE EXAMPLE

This case exemplifies points made in the chapter about the differential diagnosis of cognitive impairment in late life and the importance of background information, symptom patterns, and course of treatment. The wrong diagnosis can lead to a totally different treatment than what is needed.

Presenting Complaint
Mrs. A is an 81-year-old widow with acute onset of confusion. Her family states that for the past 2 months the patient has become increasingly irritable and forgetful. She seems unable to

recall facts or names of family and friends. She converses minimally, but when she does, she repeats herself. She complaints of feeling weak and has become afraid of falling, and now uses a walker. She neglects her personal hygiene, eats little, despite saying that her appetite is unchanged, and has had a few episodes of incontinence. The family wonders if the patient has AD.

History
The patient lost her husband 14 months ago after a prolonged illness (symptoms seem to have begun around the anniversary of his death). She apparently functioned normally for 2 months after his death, before mild depressive symptoms emerged that the family thought was expected of mourning. She was married for 61 years and in a close and supportive marriage. When prompted about her life during her husband's terminal phase, she said that she could not believe how irritable he was at the end, and how hard it was not to get mad at him.

She has a history of hypothyroidism and arthritis.

There is no prior history of depression or family history of affective disorder.

The patient is an only child. Her father died when she was 11 from an accident. She became closer to her mother, and her mother lived with her and her husband until the mother's death.

There is no family history of a psychiatric disorder, alcoholism, or dementia.

The patient had a high school education. She was a housewife and never worked professionally.

Collateral Information
The family state that the patient began to talk about loneliness shortly after her husband died. The patient had never lived alone before and was dependent upon her husband, like a stereotypical 1940s housewife. They noted that she was a good mother, but was quiet, with few friends.

MMSE = 19
Most errors were errors of omission ("I don't know") or giving up if the task was effortful, like serial 7s. The patient was oriented to time but not place. Visuospatial function and writing were intact. Remote memory seemed equally impaired as recent memory.

Medical Problems and Medications
Hypothyroidism—on Synthroid
Insomnia—occasionally takes Tylenol PM but has not for several nights

Differential Diagnoses
Axis I: *Major Depressive Disorder (296.23; major depression, moderate, first episode)*

Mood Disorder due to a general medical condition (293.83), such as hypothyroidism or stroke, must be ruled out.

Substance-Induced Mood Disorder (293.83)—unlikely here

Mood Disorder, NOS (296.90)

Dementia, NOS (294.8)

Axis II: *None*

Axis III: Hypothyroidism (treated)

Axis IV: 4 Severe—death of spouse (pathological mourning)

Axis V: Current GAF: 40—some impairment in judgment, communication, thinking and mood

Highest GAF in the past year: 70—mild symptoms

Labs and Tests
CBC (complete blood count) with differential—WNL (within normal limits)

CMP (comprehensive metabolic panel)—WNL

Thyroid panel (TSH, T4, T3-uptake)—WNL, TSH low-normal range

EKG—WNL

MRI of the brain—mild atrophy read as normal for age, with periventricular hyperintensity

Discussion
Depression in any age group is often associated with cognitive disturbance. In the elderly, the cognitive disturbance is often severe enough to appear like a dementia, causing many to call this a "pseudodementia." Depressive symptoms and cognitive disturbance can also be caused by medications such as tranquilizers or pain medications, medical illness such as hypothyroidism, stroke (over 50% of patients with anterior dominant

hemisphere CVAs develop depression), or Parkinson's disease. This is why medication history and medical review are needed.

It is widely held that core depressive symptoms such as sleep disturbance, anorexia, anhedonia, negativism, and tearfulness will persist in all major depressions and should be looked for as part of the confirmation of depression as opposed to another cause. Generally, sleep disturbance in depression fits the pattern of short sleep latency (falls asleep immediately) but interrupted sleep with early morning rising (wakes for the final time at about 4 a.m.), with concomitant daytime sleepiness.

Cognitive disturbance is generally different from Alzheimer's dementia. Usually patients with depression make errors due to "errors of omission"—they answer, "I don't know," whereas patients with dementia make "errors of commission"—they give a wrong answer. Depressed patients become low risk takers (they won't venture an answer). Depressed patients are often fully oriented but make errors on concentration tasks, such as serial subtraction, or errors on effortful tasks. Depressed patients sometimes show the reverse pattern of memory loss than in dementia, with forgetfulness of both recent and remote items, as opposed to just recent memory loss.

Depression causes an excess disability with vague symptomatology and headaches that defy symptomatic or medical treatment. In the interview, if the patient has dementia, the confusion is worse as the patient becomes more fatigued and challenged. In depression, the patient improves cognitively as the interview progresses due to engagement with the interviewer. In a secondary depression due to a medical problem or medication, symptoms wax and wane, like a delirium. Often depression occurs in dementia. Cognitive function improves but remains mildly impaired.

Atypical depression is responsive to somatic treatments for depression, both medication and ECT. It is also helped by reducing environmental stresses, helping patients develop better coping styles, and working through conflicted areas such as pathological mourning.

Patient Outcome
The patient responded well to an SSRI and psychotherapy. In this case, an SSRI was started and the patient was encouraged

to talk about her loss and future plans. A background review was the starting point of treatment. As in most cases of pseudo-dementia, the patient's cognition improved by the end of each session compared to the beginning, probably because the clinician's interest and help in working through her difficult mourning process relieved her anxiety and engaged her. No cognitive enhancers were needed. No imaging was done at the beginning, only health screening. Medications that might further impair cognitive function, namely Tylenol PM, were stopped. The patient's cognitive status returned to baseline within 3 months, accompanying remission of depressive equivalents (inattention, sleep problems, self-neglect). The patient may still develop Alzheimer's in the future, but that was not the cause of her initial disability.

SUMMARY

An accurate diagnosis of the cause of cognitive disorders in the elderly is needed to determine the optimal treatment. Nine disorders are commonly confused with one another: (1) Alzheimer's dementia, (2) Lewy body dementia, (3) frontotemporal dementia, (4) multi-infarct dementia (MID), (5) Parkinson's dementia, (6) normal pressure hydrocephalus, (7) pseudodementia (depression), (8) dementia of schizophrenia, and (9) delirium. Each disorder differs in brain localization, etiology, course, and prognosis. A brain scan helps to differentiate among them and is important, but it is only part of a standard dementia assessment. Acetylcholinesterase inhibitors are indicated for Alzheimer's dementia and Parkinson's dementia, and may be least likely to cause adverse effects in Lewy body dementia. Nonmedication interventions include memory mnemonics for mild cases and structured, failure-free activities or behavior modification techniques for the more seriously impaired. Caregiver burden must be addressed at all stages, as it can lead the patient to be prematurely institutionalized or potentially abused. Advanced directives should be addressed with the patient and family early on, and longitudinal follow-up must be provided.

4

TREATING BEHAVIORAL
DISTURBANCES ASSOCIATED
WITH DEMENTIA

Behavioral disturbances are common in neurodegenerative diseases throughout early to late stages. However, it must be emphasized that behavioral disturbances are not always present, are treatable in most instances, and although common, are not pathognomonic for any dementia. Many patients remain pleasant with only memory problems and trouble reasoning. What is called *agitation* can refer to at least 29 distinct symptoms that can be clustered into aggressive behaviors (verbal and physical) and nonaggressive behaviors (e.g., pacing or repetitive vocalizations) (Cohen-Mansfield et al., 1989). Causes may include reactions to the setting (psychosocial issues), medical discomfort, psychiatric disorders (comorbid depression, psychosis, anxiety), or an intermittent explosive disorder (impulsivity). Thus, behavioral problems are a separate issue from the cognitive impairment that defines dementia.

Gene Cohen, a former director of the Aging Branch at NIMH, was once reported to say: "Dementia is the perfect example of the Cartesian mind–body dichotomy: It is a disorder that is 100% neurological, but 100% of the symptoms are cognitive and behavioral." Dementia is often placed within the purview of psychiatry because of the behavioral manifestations. These behavioral issues have even been termed "noncognitive behaviors associated with dementia" in the U.S. literature and "behavioral and psychological symptoms of dementia" (BPSD) in the international literature.

This chapter is intended to help identify when disturbances may be amenable to psychosocial interventions, and which may require medications. It also reviews current guidelines for treatment. Although most of the recommendations are derived from studies with AD patients, they have largely been extrapolated to behavioral problems resulting from other dementias.

BACKGROUND

A longstanding view has been that there is a formal thought disorder in dementia in addition to cognitive impairment. Such psychotic symptoms include irrelevant speech, circumstantiality, logically unconnected thoughts, motor hyperactivity, mood lability, misidentification (illusions), poor judgment and insight, inability to abstract, aggression and bizarre, inappropriate behavior, auditory and visual hallucinations, and delusions (false beliefs that cannot be corrected by reason). In fact, the DSM-I and DSM-II classified dementias under psychotic disorders. Like schizophrenia, the behavioral symptoms of dementia fit both positive symptom clusters (hallucinations, delusions, aggression, bizarre and inappropriate affect and behavior) and negative symptoms (apathy, anhedonia [no pleasure], avolition [no will], paucity of ideation [mind is blank] and paucity of speech).

Neurobiological Explanation

There are no animal models for agitation in dementia. Biological assumptions about symptom causation consider similarities to other psychiatric diagnoses. It is assumed that serotonin and norepinephrine system dysregulation may underlie aggression and depressive symptoms; GABA or glutamate dysregulation and abnormalities underlie psychomotor agitation and anxiety; acetylcholine system dysregulation underlies apathy and confusion; and dopamine system dysregulation, acetylcholine, and serotonin all underlie psychosis. These assumptions have treatment implications for the selection of medications, which will be addressed the treatment section (McShane, 2000).

Proof of efficacy of medications or behavioral approaches for agitation should be established from double-blind placebo-controlled studies or comparisons between two treatments. However, studies of treatments for agitation in dementia remain sparse because of diagnostic heterogeneity (different causes for the dementia) and because agitation encompasses so many symptoms and causes. That is, it is not a clear-cut syndrome.

Psychosis in dementia requires special attention because it may have a different mechanism than schizophrenia. The pattern of psychosis and characteristic symptoms differ. For example, in AD there is often immediate, rather than delayed, responsiveness in psychotic symptoms to antipsychotic medications; effective doses of the antipsychotic are lower; and AChEIs often resolve mild psychotic symptoms. Psychosis in AD rarely entails complex delusions, often involves visual hallucinations, rarely has associated suicidal ideation, and waxes and wanes more (e.g., absent during the day, only present at night). Caregiver misidentification is common, and there is rarely a past history of psychosis (Jeste & Finkel, 2000). A cholinergic model for psychosis was proposed in which the low acetylcholine function seen in AD and some dementias may be similar to an anticholinergic psychosis from medications (Cummings & Back, 1998).

NORMAL VERSUS ABNORMAL BEHAVIOR

There is a longstanding opposing view to the biological model that behavioral disorders are merely due to pathological coping due to cognitive impairment. Patients with cognitive impairment act in very childlike ways—that is, they show distractibility, poor capacity for effective self-regulation in the face of stress (affective flooding), and use of "primitive or immature defenses" (mainly denial, acting out, or projection). They also show the inappropriate coping style of acting first and questioning later, or never questioning. Because of these deficits, the patient seems overwhelmed by the least stress or change and reacts to every change or conflict as a catastrophe (catastrophic reaction), with agitation, changes in mood, screaming, crying, and verbal and physical aggression (Alzheimer's Disease Resource Agency, 2004). Coping styles appear "primitive" and impulsive, free of reason. It is like the proverbial "fire–ready–aim" sequence of behavior, rather than the rational and recommended "ready–aim–fire" sequence.

One observation has been that the loss of function that comes with dementia follows a reverse pattern from child development, which could be called "a trip back in time" (Johnson, 2000). This trip is not reversible because it is not a psychological defensive regression to stress, and it must be managed through environmental supports—milieu therapy. From a psychiatric vantage point, it is useful to recall the hierarchy of defenses first proposed by Anna Freud (1937), which was empirically validated by Vaillant and his colleagues (1986) in normal adults (see Table 4.1). It is evident that the most mature and adaptive defensive styles—intellectualization, humor, and sublimation—are no longer available to dementia patients, whereas the earliest and most primitive styles of denial, projection (blaming others), and acting out (temper tantrums or immediate gratification) are. As in child development, this hierarchy predicts which level of interaction and coping capacity a dementia patient might still posses. The table is useful to review with caregivers to help dispel their expectation that a dementia patient should act like an adult and not cause conflict. Many families, and even staff, wrongfully interpret these primitive reactive styles as passive–aggressive behavior meant to deliberately irritate. Recognition of the return of these childlike reactions to stress allows one to respond in a more understanding way, without anger or irritation. If the cause of behavioral disturbances is nonbiological, then supervision and structure would be preferable to medications.

Table 4.1. Hierarchy of Defenses

PREDOMINATE IN DEMENTIA AGAIN

Developmentally early/psychotic defenses
- Denial (unconscious; no awareness)
- Projection (blaming; attributes feelings to someone else in the external world)

Immature defenses
- Acting out (direct expression of wishes, impulses, and fantasies)
- Dissociation
- Regression (they do not feel they have to act in mature and responsible ways)

UNAVAILABLE TO THE DEMENTIA PATIENT

Neurotic defenses
- Repression (involves complete forgetting)
- Reaction formation (a "bad" wish becomes a "good" one)
- Displacement (wishes are directed away from one person and redirected toward another)
- Undoing (acting in ways that symbolically make amends)

Table 4.1. (continued)

Mature defenses
- Sublimation (finds alternative gratification pathway)
- Humor (nonoffensive way to express painful or otherwise unacceptable wishes and feelings)

Source: Adapted from Valliant (1992).

It has also been a longstanding assumption that nonverbal communication must replace normal speech in aphasic and dementia patients. The concept of symbolic speech, or latent meaning, must be revived in making inferences from behavioral patterns. The patients themselves are usually unaware of what they want to say, so correctness of interpretations is determined by improvement in patient behavior or subsequent relevant communication after one guesses at the correct intervention. Naomi Feil developed her validation technique for patients with AD around this view. First described in 1963, the technique uses an intuitive approach of what the patient might be trying to say, starting with an assumption that all behavior is meaningful and validating patients' implied needs or feelings with direct gratification (i.e., doing what you think they want) or rephrasing what you think they are trying to communicate to show that you understand. This approach has been effective in reducing agitation (Feil, 2002) and can be applied to any patient who lacks insight or the capacity for verbal communication, including regressed psychotic patients. An additional communication principle for caregivers is to introduce their intent verbally before acting. For example, countless conflicts over bathing could be eliminated by caregivers letting patients know that they are preparing the bath and will be back to help them in a few minutes. An additional aid: Post a schedule to which patients can refer.

UNIQUE ASPECTS OF AGITATION IN ELDERLY

The behavioral disturbance associated with dementia is considered a separate entity under Medicare. If records are audited, diagnostic codes that correspond to agitation or a primary psychiatric disorder must be present to justify treatment. This is especially true for inpatient psychiatric hospitalization. DSM-IV-TR codes that relate to agitation are given in Table 4.2.

Table 4.2. DSM-IV Diagnoses for Behavioral
Disturbances Associated with Dementia

Dementia with Behavioral Disturbance	294.11

SAMPLE CAUSES FOR THE BEHAVIORAL DISTURBANCE:

Major Depression	296.3x
Bipolar Disorder (relatively rare phenomenon)	296.5x, 296.6x
Psychotic Disorder NOS	289.9
Delusional Disorder	297.1
Anxiety Disorder NOS	300.00
Delirium Due to . . .	293.0
Delirium NOS	780.09
Adjustment Disorder with Disturbance of Conduct	309.3
Intermittent Explosive Disorder	312.34
Impulse Control Disorder NOS	312.30

Note. Any of the above diagnoses can be applied if the clinician believes that the psychiatric diagnoses are comorbid conditions rather than directly due to the general medical condition, such as AD, or other demonstrable organic or personality disorder that better accounts for the behavior. General rules to determine comorbid conditions are:

- *Symptoms persist when cognition improves.*
- *Occurrence is temporally linked to occurrence of a psychosocial precipitant.*
- *There is a preexisting psychiatric diagnosis that may have recurred.*
- *Symptoms seem to wax and wane.*

ASSESSMENT AND DIAGNOSIS

Both the behavioral and neurobiological models have implications for treatment. The biological model suggests medications and the psychological coping model suggests behavioral management. Both are applicable for different situations, and neither approach can be universally applied.

The major psychological causes are:

- Episodic reaction with a temporal association to an interpersonal argument
- Episodic, with a temporal association to a psychosocial stressor (loss, move, other worry)
- Excessive stimulation levels (noise, too much going on in the home)
- Too little stimulation level (boredom)

The major biological causes are:

- Physical discomfort (usually pain or condition causing delirium)
- No clear psychosocial precipitants
- Relatively constant behaviors or behaviors that show an intrinsic diurnal pattern, such as sundowning

Table 4.3 summarizes the types of behavioral disturbances in dementia.

Table 4.3. Types of Behavioral Disturbances in Dementia

UNDERLYING ETIOLOGY	FINDINGS	BEHAVIORAL OBSERVATIONS
Primary neurobiological cause (may need medication)	Diurnal rhythm (e.g., sundowning), constant agitation, insomnia, generalized aggression (mad at everyone and everything)	Usually no psychosocial precipitant
Primary psychiatric diagnosis	Depression, psychotic disorder, anger directed at delusional object for no apparent reason	Difficult to diagnose due to speech and insight impairment; often inferred from behavior (e.g., talking to self, crying, not eating, fear of others)

Table 4.3. (continued)

Primary reactive cause (need behavioral intervention)	Immediately follows some stress; patient reacts negatively to only one person; aggression directed at one person following some grievance	Usually behavioral interventions are best; the patient tends to be overwhelmed easily (affective flooding), shows poor self-regulation (impulsivity) and distractibility
Unknown cause	Pacing, repetitious speech or questions	Usually behavioral interventions are best, such as redirection, distraction, music/entertainment, "play"

Insomnia has many causes, and may respond to behavioral interventions (no stimulants or naps) or medications at other times. This area is addressed in Chapter 8.

Identification of depression in advanced dementia requires special comment because of the absence of insight or verbal abilities in most patients. A relatively short scale, the Cornell Scale of Depression in Dementia (Alexopoulos et al., 1988), based on observations instead of verbal complaints, is often useful as a tool to codify staff and personal observations for patients without insight into their feelings. This is a 38-point scale, reproduced in Table 4.4, wherein 12 or higher is usually indicative of major depression.

Table 4.4. Cornell Scale of Depression in Dementia

MOOD-RELATED SIGNS
1. Anxious expression, rumination, worrying
2. Sad expression, sad voice, tearfulness
3. Lack of reaction to pleasant events
4. Annoyed and short tempered

BEHAVIORAL DISTURBANCES
1. Restless, hand wringing, hair pulling
2. Psychomotor retardation—slow movements, slow speech, slow reactions
3. Multiple physical complaitns
4. Loss of interest and withdrawal from usual activities

Table 4.4 (continued)

PHYSICAL SIGNS
1. Eating less than usual
2. Weight loss
3. Fatigues easily, no energy

CYCLIC FUNCTIONS
1. Diurnal mood variation
2. Difficulty with sleep (early, middle, or late insomnia)

IDEATIONAL DISTURBANCE
1. Feels life is not worth living
2. Poor self-esteem with feelings of failure, self-blame, or self-depreciation
3. Anticipates the worst, pessimistic
4. Mood-congruent delusions—delusions of poverty (e.g., refuses help because can't afford it), delusions of illness (e.g., always calling for the doctor), delusions of loss (e.g., a family member has just died)

Note. A copy can be downloaded from www.emoryhealthcare.org/departments/fuqua/CornellScale.pdf.

TREATMENT METHODS

Behavioral symptoms that respond best to medication are manifestations of psychiatric disorders such as depression or psychosis, or of aggression and nonrandom motoric hyperactivity, such as:

- Behavioral symptoms with a clear diurnal pattern
- Impulsive aggression (not temper tantrums when one doesn't get one's way)
- Behavioral symptoms well above "normal"—exaggerated response

Behavioral symptoms that respond best to behavioral interventions are nonaggressive behaviors such as:

- Pacing
- Perseveration (speech or behavior)
- Appropriating
- Catastrophic reactions to minor environmental changes

- Inappropriate social behaviors
- Toileting problems (e.g., going in the wastebasket, smearing feces)
- Repetitive vocalizations (e.g., grunting, screaming)
- Inability to delay gratification

Medications

There are no approved medications for behavioral disturbances associated with dementia. Antipsychotics are approved for schizophrenia and bipolar illness, but not for psychosis related to AD. Table 4.5 lists categories of current off-label prescribing recommendations tabulated from consensus panels. When psychosis is present, the first choice is a novel antipsychotic. An alternative for mild psychotic symptoms in AD patients (ideation only, not acting out the psychosis) is starting an AChEI first because this class of drugs seems to reduce behavioral disturbances as well as improve cognition (Lavretsky & Nguyen, 2006).

Table 4.5. Choice of Medication by Target Symptom

APATHY
    AChE inhibitors
    Antidepressants

AGGRESSION
    Antipsychotics
    Anticonvulsants
    Antidepressants

PSYCHOMOTOR AGITATION
    Antipsychotics
    Anticonvulsants
    Benzodiazepines
    Antidepressants

PSYCHOSIS
    Antipsychotics
    AChE inhibitors

DEPRESSION
    Antidepressants

Source: Adapted from McShane (2000); Brodaty & Finkel (2003).

Geriatric dose ranges are highly subjective, but the "dementia range" is usually about 50% of usual adult doses as shown in Table 4.6.

Table 4.6. Geriatric Dose Ranges for Dementia

	Starting Dose	Target Dose
ANTIPSYCHOTICS		
Aripiprazole (Abilify)	2.5 or 5 mg/day	10–15 mg/day
Clozapine (Clozaril)	12.5 mg/day	50–200 mg/day
Haloperidol (Haldol)	0.25–0.5 mg/day	2–5 mg/day
Olanzepine (Zyprexa, Zydis)	2.5–5 mg/day	10–15 mg/day
Quetiapine (Seroquel)	25–50 mg/day	100–400 mg/day
Risperidone (Risperdal)	0.25–0.5 mg/day	0.5–1.0 mg/day
Ziprasidone (Geodon)	10–20 mg/day	20–40 mg/day
MOOD STABILIZERS AND ANTICONVULSANTS		
Carbamazepine (Tegretol)	100 mg qd or bid	400 mg/day or antileptic level 4–12 mg/mL
Gabapentin (Neurontin)	100 mg/day	600–1200 mg/day
Lamotrigine	25–50 mg/day	150–400 mg/day
Lithium	150 mg/day	titrate to 0.4–0.8 meq/L
Valproic acid	125–250 mg/day	500 mg/day or antileptic level 50–120 mg/L)
MOOD STABILIZERS WITH THEORETICAL VALUE DUE TO ANXIOLYTIC EFFECT		
Pregabalin (Lyrica)	25–50 mg/day	100 mg bid
Oxycarbazepine (Trileptal)	150 mg qd or bid	500 mg/day
Levetiracetam (Keppra)	500 mg qd	1000 mg qd
BENZODIAZEPINES		
Lorazepam	0.25–0.5 mg prn	1–3 mg/day in divided doses
Oxazepam	5.0–7.5 mg prn	5.0–7.5 mg/day in divided doses
Alprazolam	Generally not used for this indication due to amnestic effects and dependency potential	

Table 4.6. (continued)

CHOLINESTERASE INHIBITORS

Donepezil (Aricept)	5 mg qd	10 mg qd
Galantamine (Razadyne)	4 mg bid with meals	12 mg bid with meals
Rivastigmine (Exelon)	1.5 mg bid with meals	6 mg bid with meals

Not studied for this indication. Source: Adapted from Cheong (2004).

Which medication should be used first is also an individual preference since there are no approved medications. One widely quoted study with risperidone (Katz et al., 1999) showed cognitive impairment and extrapyramidal side effects (EPS) above 2 mg/day, with even more noticeable side effects with equivalent doses of haloperidol. Although efficacy of haloperidol and risperidone were essentially equal in the Katz study, a more recent head-to-head comparison of risperidone versus haloperidol for agitation in dementia showed significantly improved efficacy with the atypical antipsychotic (risperidone; Suh et al., 2006).

To address these issues, a head-to-head comparison between novel antipsychotic medications for psychosis in AD was supported by NIMH. The recently completed Clinical Antipsychotic Trials of Intervention Effectiveness—Alzheimer's Disease (CATIE-AD) trial did not show significant differences in efficacy, but in terms of median time to discontinuation of treatment, risperidone and olanzapine were favored (possibly best tolerated; Schneider et al., 2006). Quetiapine was added to the study later, but aripiprazole was launched too late to be added until the third tier (after failure of two medications). Although the use of any antipsychotic is off-label in dealing with agitation associated with delirium or dementia, atypical antipsychotics offer the advantage of causing less confusion and fewer EPS that could cause falls, and is still the medication preferred by most geriatric psychiatrists (Alexopoulos et al., 2005).

There is a current FDA black-box warning about excess mortality in patients with dementia treated with atypical antipsychotics. In a meta-analysis of studies totaling 3,353

patients randomized to study medication and 1,757 randomized to placebo, the odds ratio was 1.54 higher deaths compared to placebo (Schneider, 2005). A similar finding was
found in elderly VA populations who were treated with antipsychotic medication (Hollis et al., 2006). No causal relationship
or mechanism could be determined from a review of the literature. A minority opinion of geriatric psychiatrists is that even
the relatively low increase in risk of stroke or sudden death in
dementia patients treated with second-generation antipsychotics (atypicals) (black box warning) outweighs any potential
benefits (Ames et al., 2005). Typical (older) antipsychotics are
not well tolerated on other grounds. Because of limited treatment alternatives for psychosis or severe agitation, both the
American Association for Geriatric Psychiatry (AAGP) and
International Psychogeriatric Association (IPA) advocate off-
label use of antipsychotics if done judiciously and with
informed consent from the families about the black-box warning (American Association for Geriatric Psychiatry, 2005). The
principles outlined in Chapter 2 should be followed to avoid
polypharmacy and to assure that lower doses are used to
increase safety.

Choice of the initial medication is often based on secondary
health factors or sedative potential of a medication. As a group,
the antipsychotics are effective in 61% of patients, compared
with 35% placebo, in reducing agitation (Cheong, 2004). The
atypical antipsychotics are preferred over conventional antipsychotics such as haloperidol because of markedly lower rates
of tardive dyskinesia (Jeste et al., 2000), parkinsonism, and
confusion.

The CATIE-AD trial used the following starting doses: quetiapine 25 mg, risperidone 0.5 mg, and olanzepine 2.5 mg.
Dose adjustments were allowed every 2 weeks for 12 weeks. If
a patient did not respond, he or she was randomly assigned to
one of the other antipsychotics or citalopram 5 mg at similar
starting doses, with dose adjustment allowed every 2 weeks for
another 12 weeks. Citalopram was used because SSRIs are
thought to reduce aggression and impulsivity as well as weakly
blocking dopamine for mild antipsychotic action. The maximum doses allowed were: quetiapine 200 mg/day, risperidone

2.0 mg/day, olanzepine 10 mg/day, and citalopram 30 mg/day. Ziprasidone and aripiprazole were not available when the trial was conducted.

In terms of theoretical preference when the following comorbid diseases are present:

- Quetiapine is the first choice in patients with Parkinson's who are on Sinemet because it has the least dopamine (D2) receptor occupancy at therapeutic doses and the least negative impact on PD symptoms.
- Aripiprazole may be first choice in PD patients who are not on Sinemet or for patients with Lewy body dementia, because it is a partial agonist that acts as either a dopamine antagonist or agonist, based on regional dopamine.
- Ziprasidone may be the first choice in patients where intramuscular (IM) medication is required or low sedation is required.
- Ziprasidone is not indicated in patients with significant QTc prolongation, recent acute myocardial infarction, uncompensated heart failure, cardiac arrhythmia, or who are at risk for significant electrolyte imbalance (from package insert).
- Olanzapine or quetiapine may be the medication of choice if sedation is required.
- Olanzapine may be a late choice if there is preexisting diabetes or obesity.
- Haloperidol may be a first choice with delirium because prolonged exposure is not usually needed.
- Haloperidol is not a good choice for extended use because of the risk of tardive dyskinesia and EPS.
- Clozapine is always reserved for treatment-resistant cases due to the risk of agranulocytosis and seizures and the inconvenience of frequent WBC monitoring.
- Intermediate-acting low-dose benzodiazepines, such as lorazepam or alprazolam, are even used in clinical trials as a "rescue medication" while dose titration is underway.
- Caution should always be exercised in using benzodiazepines with frail dementia patients because the medication may cause a paradoxical excitement, confusion, or falls.

In all cases, dose titration is needed. Push to optimal efficacy or maximum allowed doses.

It is also important to emphasize the geriatric principles described in Chapter 2 regarding sequential, single medication trials rather than polypharmacy, and to "start low, go slow, but go." The speed of titration depends upon patient tolerance. Push the dose quickly to what is thought to be the target dose, and then continue to increase more slowly at five half-life intervals, to avoid accumulation effects and toxicity.

Psychosocial Interventions

Management of behavioral problems is relatively nonspecific. Behavioral interventions generally involve one of the following:

- Stimulus reduction (time out, shutting off the TV, soft music)
- Removing a psychosocial stress that is causing pathological reactions
- Distraction
- Behavioral modification (rewarding appropriate behaviors through praise or social rewards, but avoid punishing negative behaviors)
- Reassurance and support (be an alter-ego for the patient, like a maternal figure who can provide whatever the patient cannot do him- or herself)
- Trying to understand and respond to latent meanings of nonverbal communications

Effectiveness of such interventions appears to be modest. Cohen-Mansfield (2001) reviewed 83 studies of psychosocial interventions alone for approaches used and efficacy. Although these studies were all performed in institutional settings, it is important to teach caregivers, families, and staff the basic models employed by these studies. When done correctly, small-group settings, rather than intensive individual sessions, are less stressful and more effective for many patients with dementia. The range of behavioral interventions that have been used with dementia patients is listed in Table 4.7.

Table 4.7. Psychosocial Interventions for Dementia

SENSORY STIMULATION
- Massage, caring touch
- Manicures
- Music—often played during meals and bathing (times of peak agitation)
  - Quiet music, classical music, or favorites (e.g., "oldies")
  - Individualized music tapes
  - White noise audiotapes (surf, environmental sounds)
- Music therapy (singing, playing instruments, music games)
- Aromatherapy

COGNITIVE INTERVENTIONS/COMMUNICATION/
ONE-TO-ONE INTERACTION
- Side conversation, distraction
- Reality orientation
- Validation therapy
- Problem solving

BEHAVIOR THERAPY (CONDITIONED LEARNING, NOT
COGNITIVE—BEHAVIORAL THERAPY)
- Differential reinforcement (usually food or praise) for "quiet behavior"
- Skill elicitation (habit training, ADL assistance)
- Spaced retrieval training (e.g., associate a cue with the location of the toilet)

STIMULUS CONTROL
- Reduced stimulation
- Environmental cues (e.g., place mirrors in front of exit doors)
- General milieu changes
- Two-dimensional grid pattern on the floor to redirect
- Verbal or physical prompts
- Disguise door or place visual barrier in front of it
- Environmental modifications (e.g., stop signs, orienting cues, lighting, predictable routines)
- Corridors decorated uniquely

SOCIAL ACTIVITIES OR CUES
- Videotapes of family (supplied by family)
- Simulated presence (tape-recorded message from the family)
- Pet therapy/companion animals
- Interactive videotapes
- Individualized activities (patient preference)
- Communication/problem-solving strategy
- New routine
- Outdoor walks

Table 4.7. (continued)

STRUCTURED UNIT ACTIVITIES
- Increase daytime activities (e.g., relaxation training, reminiscence therapy, word games, crafts)
- Special programs (entertainers)
- Therapeutic trips
- Recreational activities (e.g., sorting, sewing, manipulating)
- Phototherapy

PHYSICAL ACTIVITIES
- Sensorimotor programs
- Exercise

MISCELLANEOUS INTERVENTIONS
- Bright light therapy (exposure to at least 1 hour/day of 1,500–2000 lux—bright daylight equivalent)
- Pain management
- Hearing aids
- Remove restraints

STAFF TRAINING
- Empathy training
- Skill training
- Theory training
- Review psychiatric medications
- Educational rounds

Note. ADL-activities of daily living. Source: Adapted from Cohen-Mansfield (2001) and Alexopoulos et al. (2005).

It is also often helpful to teach communication strategies to families. The skills involve simplifying verbal language to patients' level of understanding for the cognitively impaired, and using nonverbal or written forms of communication for aphasic patients. As with the development of any clinical skill, training involves cognitive information (from teaching and reading), modeling (caregivers observe clinician), and supervision (clinician observes interactions and corrects). Table 4.8 presents a summary of recommended communication strategies.

Table 4.8. Recommended Communication
Strategies

1. Use short, simple sentences.
2. Speak slowly.
3. Ask one question at a time or present sequential instructions one step at a
   time.
4. Avoid interrupting the patient.
5. Allow plenty of time for patient response.
6. Establish eye contact and approach slowly from the front rather than the
   back.
7. Eliminate distractions (shut off the TV or radio while
   communicating).
8. Use yes/no rather than open-ended questions.
9. Paraphrase repeated messages that the patient may not
   understand.
10. Use the same wording when repeating messages that are
    understood.
11. Ask the patient to talk around the word for which he or she is searching
    (describe it or describe the context; circumlocution).
12. Use visual cues (patients often point to what they want or
    mean).
13. Be aware of paraphasias (word substitutions by the patient).
14. Make topic context bound (e.g., speak about food preferences when eating,
    not in between meals).
15. Use distraction or change the subject if a topic is upsetting to the patient
    (i.e., if he or she is getting agitated); come back to the topic later, when the
    patient is calmer.

Source: Adapted and amplified (nos. 12–15) from Small & Gutman (2002).

A strategy that has been widely adopted by professionals in the
fields of nursing and social work is validation therapy (Feil, 2002).
The worker verbally rephrases the apparent meaning of nonverbal
communications or less meaningful verbal attempts by the patient
and asks if that is correct, then directly gratifies the patient's needs
when known (validation). Agitation is reduced if the patient feels
understood and his or her needs are met, as attested to by adher-
ents of this treatment (Day, 1997).

Table 4.9 summarizes behavioral treatment selections for management of agitation in patients with dementia.

Table 4.9. Intervention Grid for Management
of Agitation in Dementia

MEDICAL	PSYCHIATRIC	FEAR/ANXIETY
Medical Interventions		
Treat causes of delirium	Ensure compliance with	Consider appropriate
Assess for medication side	appropriate psy-	psychotropic medica-
effects	chotropic medication	tion
	Provide supportive psy-	Possibly add AD medica-
	chotherapy if patient is	tion
	capable	
Psychosocial Interventions		
Limit distractions	Facilitate reorientation	Facilitate orientation (ori-
Provide quiet environ-	Similar environmental	ent to new setting)
ment or soft music	considerations to med-	Provide quiet environ-
Have a family attendant	ical causes	ment or soft music
for reassurance	Provide explanations and	Use family attendant for
Install a bed alarm if fall	reassurance	reassurance
risk	Encourage group activi-	Use calm, nonthreatening
Use calm, nonthreatening	ties	approach
approach	Maintain consistent	Allow familiar possessions
Provide explanations and	schedule	Provide explanations and
reassurance	Avoid stimulants at night	reassurance

A Final Note

Psychiatric hospitalization for patients with dementia generally occurs only for severe agitation or violence to self or others. Each discipline on the treatment team should strive to
complete its evaluation portion within the first 48 hours of
admission because of the usual limitations for insurance coverage. Table 4.10 provides a summary of evaluations and treatments needed, by discipline, for hospitalized patients with
dementia.

Table 4.9. (continued)

DISCOMFORT	BOREDOM	SLEEP PROBLEM
Medical Interventions		
Provide pain management	Order appropriate involvements	Diagnose sleep disorder or psychiatric cause
Order laxatives		Administer hypnotics if indicated
Assess full bladder		
Order positioning		
Hydrate/feed		
Psychosocial Interventions		
Provide quiet environment or soft music	Provide activities therapy	Prevent daytime napping
Provide explanations and reassurance	Provide socialization	Avoid stimulants at night
	Provide occupational therapy	Ensure toilet use before sleep
	Provide reminiscence therapy	Provide quiet environment
		Maintain consistent schedule
		Replicate home bedtime schedule
		Provide soft music or relaxation before sleep

SUMMARY

Behavioral disturbances that occur in more than half of patients with dementia may be a reflection of inappropriate coping, but also may be due to intrinsic brain changes that require medications to address psychosis, mood disorders, generalized anxiety, aggression, or nonspecific diurnal changes. In practice, behavioral management approaches should be tried before medications unless there are clear-cut signs of psychosis or depression. Care providers must also learn how to recognize and accommodate dementia-related changes in a patient's speech or self-care. With all psychotropic medications, unwanted confusion and paradoxical increases in agitation can occur if there are further compromises of thought processes.

Table 4.10. Interdisciplinary Inpatient Evaluation and Treatment
Responsibilities for Behavioral Disturbance

PSYCHIATRY	NURSING
Psychiatric evaluation	ADL assessment (evaluate reversibility)
Neurological screening	Nursing assessment (medical needs)
Mental status examination	Send for collateral records
Review records	Administer medications
Obtain prior psych meds history and doses	Monitor sleep, social participation, intake
Order and review tests	Provide medical education
Establish DSM-IV diagnosis	Lead groups
Categorize target symptoms (type, frequency, severity, cause)	Assess social appropriateness and readiness for discharge
Coordinate care with other disciplines	
Order and monitor psychotropic medications	
Provide psychotherapy	

Benzodiazepines are most likely to cause falls and confusion and
should be used cautiously, if at all. Novel antipsychotic medications
have fewer side effects but all have a black box warning about
slightly higher mortality rates, and many are associated with an
increase in a metabolic syndrome (increased appetite, weight gain,
and insulin resistance). The goal in treating behavioral disturbances
related to dementia is usually to reduce the frequency and severity
of problems; rarely is total elimination of the disturbance possible.

Table 4.10. (continued)

OCCUPATIONAL THERAPY	SOCIAL WORK
Functional testing (IADL)	Family contact for collateral information on course, current functioning, and social supports
Executive function assessment	
Assess awareness of risks	
Assess ability to communicate needs	Network assessment (genogram, ecomap, caregiver burden)
Assess social appropriateness	
Lead groups	Care counseling
Establish repertoire of behavioral strategies for outpatient caregivers	Provide resource information
	Maintain knowledge of community resources (day care, home health, housing, nursing homes, self-help groups)
Assess if able to communicate needs	
	Provide links to outside programs and services
	Lead patient and family groups
	Advise about advanced directive and legal needs

5

MOOD DISORDERS

Diagnostic categories for geriatric depression use the same DSM-IV-TR categories as general adults. Mood disorders typically encompass the following:

- Major depression (first episode 296.2, recurrent epidose 296.3)
- Bipolar mood disorders (single manic episode 296.0, hypo-manic or manic 296.4, depressed 296.5, mixed 296.6, unspecified 296.7 or 296.80, and Bipolar II 296.89)
- Dysthymic disorder (300.4)
- Cyclothymic disorder (301.13) (rarely seen in elderly)
- Mood disorders due to a medical condition or substance-induced (293.83)
- Mood disorder not otherwise specified (atypical depression)

Elderly patients suffering from a subtype of unipolar depression often present with atypical symptoms because depression in this population often looks different from depression in younger patients, and is frequently associated with underlying vascular or medical causes. Similarly, the manifestation of bipolar mood disorders in older patients are often different from mania seen in younger patients due to a higher rate of "secondary mania," which is caused by an underlying neurological disease and substance use, including prescription medicines. Awareness of these different presentations is needed to effectively direct treatment. The main risk with depression in the elderly is suicide. Correlates of increased baseline risk for suicide are commonly taught, but the clinician must be aware of imminent signs of suicide to determine when to hospitalize. ECT remains the traditional approach for treatment-resistant affective disorder and psychosis, with an 80% remission rate in even in the most refractory cases. Its mechanism of action has been elucidated in experimental epilepsy studies and we now better understand the ways in which it reduces cognitive impairment.

Community studies find 25% of elderly persons reporting mild depressive symptoms, but major depression occurs at a similar rate in younger adults at 1% to 9% (Steffens, Skoog, Norton et al., 2000). Geriatric depression is highest in those who are medically ill, suffer from dementia, or have just experienced a stroke.

DEPRESSION

Background

Depression is a major cause of emotional suffering in older adults, but it often remains underdiagnosed or misdiagnosed. The first Consensus Development Conference on Geriatric Depression by NIH in 1991 highlighted the problem. It countered the commonly held opinion at the time that depression in late life is an expectable reaction to loss and change associated with age, rather than a disorder similar to major depression in younger adults. Although this view is no longer widely held, identifying and understanding depression in older adults often seems different because patients may be preoccupied with confusion, anergy, sleep disturbances, pain, or physical aspects of depression. Depressive symptoms secondary to a medical illness such as hypothyroidism or as a medication side effect are also seen more commonly.

In a medical outcome study of primary care practice, a depression screening instrument was given to 634 patients within a fixed timeframe. Then a Diagnostic Interview Schedule was administered to all subjects with positive screens for major depression, and psychotropic medication type and dose were reviewed as a proxy for appropriate treatment—because an antidepressant trial is considered the standard of care if major depression were indicated on screening. No treatment was found in 58% of patients with major depression. Of those treated, 23% were on antidepressants alone or with a minor tranquilizer, 19% were on a minor tranquilizer alone, and of those on antidepressants, only 26% were on therapeutic doses (Wells et al., 1994).

Demographically, more women than men are depressed in younger age groups by a 2:1 ratio. However, more elderly men also get depressed, making the gender disparity less pronounced with age.

Neurobiological Explanation

The catecholamine theory of depression has dominated since the 1950s, when reserpine, an antihypertensive, was found to cause depression in a large number of cases. Serotonin and norepinephrine dysfunction have been implicated as the main causal association with depression. However, it is increasingly clear that vascular risk factors and striatofrontal dysfunction are also related to geriatric depression. For example, 20–50% of patients with stroke develop depression in the first year, and there is an extremely high rate of "silent strokes" found on imaging in older adults with depression, leading to speculations that vascular causes may underlie many geriatric depressions (American Association for Geriatric Psychiatry, 2005). Subcortical ischemic change, reflected in increased white matter hyperintensities and due to interruption in normal neuronal pathways within the limbic system, is the most common associated feature of geriatric depression (Alexopoulos, 2003; Alexopoulos et al., 1997). Dysfunction in the hypothalamic–pituitary–(HPA) axis is seen in many disease states as well, and seems to play a major role in depression.

Medications that contribute to depression often involve catecholamine inhibition, hormonal effects, or effects on the HPA axis. Table 5.1 lists the medications most commonly associated with depression in older adults in approximate strength of effect.

Table 5.1. Medications Commonly Associated with Depression

α-methyldopa	Estrogen
Reserpine	Progesterone
Propranalol	Tamoxifen
Clonidine	Cimetidine
Hydralazine	Digitalis
Benzodiazepines	Vinblastine
Corticosteroids	Vincristine

Normal versus Abnormal Behavior

Patients often deemphasize affective complaints and overemphasize health or other nonaffective issues. Many older adults believe that the physical manifestations of depression (i.e., the neurovegetative depressive features) represent a physical illness. Symptoms such as anergy, insomnia, appetite change, and mild cognitive change occur with many disease states other than depression, so it is also easy for a clinician to misinterpret these features. However, somatic preoccupations, confusion, or excess disability in the presence of relatively stable health suggests depression.

Clinicians frequently do not probe for specific depressive symptoms, instead waiting for patients to volunteer information. Given physicians' time constraints, there may be insufficient time to explore symptoms or think about the incongruity between relatively mild objective findings and excessive complaints or disability. When patients call their physicians about pain, headaches, fatigue, insomnia, gastrointestinal symptoms, arthritis, weight loss, or diffuse somatic symptoms, it is common to think of the patient as being hypochondriacal rather than depressed.

Most cases of suspected depression in older adults would meet DSM-IV criteria for a major depression if symptoms were not automatically discounted as medical problems.

Unique Aspects of the Disorder in Elderly

Geriatric depression is associated with functional decline, cognitive loss, excess disability, pain, and poor health outcomes. Spontaneous remission appears to be less common in late-life depression as well, although older adults do respond to treatment at rates as high as those for younger adults.

Mild depression that persists for several years (dysthymia, 300.4) occurs frequently in elderly people. Subsyndromal depression is not actually a diagnostic category but suggests even less severe symptomatology or shorter duration than dysthymia. These minor symptoms may be due to chronic worries about money, health, safety, or grief, the condition is more akin to what used to be called "existential depression" or "common, everyday misery" (adjustment disorder with depressed mood, 309.0).

Efficacy of antidepressant medication treatment for dysthymia and subsyndromal depression remains unproven.

Assessment and Diagnosis

The only way for a clinician to improve diagnosis is to spend more time in the diagnostic process sorting out complexities, reviewing concomitant medications, and reviewing the severity of medical diagnoses. Sensitive biological markers for subtypes of depression do not yet exist.

Atypical depression is often labeled "depression without sadness." Core depressive features of anhedonia or apathy, sleep disturbance (usually hypersomnia), social withdrawal, anorexia, and psychomotor retardation are present, although typically attributed to medical problems by the patient. Even social withdrawal is described in different terms. Patients often state that they want to go out but are just too sick to enjoy themselves or feel too tired. In other words, the core depressive symptoms can be recognized if the clinician temporarily suspends judgment on the source of the symptoms. Memory complaints in pseudodementia are classically errors of indifference ("I don't know" answers), inattention, or ambivalence (cannot decide), rather than a true dementia. The common "atypical presentations" of depression are listed in Table 5.2.

Table 5.2. Common Atypical Presentations of Depression in Older Adults

TYPE OF ATYPICAL DEPRESSION	FEATURES
Secondary Mood Disorder Due to a nonpsychiatric medical condition (e.g., anergy and distress related to uremia, CHF, arrhythmias, CNS medications, hypothyroidism, neurological diseases, cancer, infections, chronic pain, and other less common etiologies)	Generally no psychiatric precipitant or life stress is reported; symptoms appear congruent with severity of physical distress.
Substance-Induced Mood Disorder Occurs while intoxicated or during withdrawal. With older adults substances of abuse are often prescribed medications rather than illicit drugs.	Although usually temporally linked, some instances persist for days but are initiated by substance use.

Table 5.2. (continued)

Masked Depression

Characterized by a subjective experience of discomfort ("I just feel bad") with motor agitation or slowing, pessimism, fear, ruminative thinking, decreased concentration, difficulty initiating action, excessive searching for medical assistance, and a denial of mood disturbance.

Usually there is a history of past depression, and denial and avoidance are presumed as primary psychological defense.

Depressive Equivalents

Borrowed from the child literature to capture conversion-like reactions. GI complaints, headaches, and a variety of somatiform symptoms are viewed as depression instead of hypochondriasis or other somatiform disorder. No clear differentiating criteria between somatization and depression have been developed, although neurovegetative depressive features are characteristic of depression.

Some instances are related to presumed conversion reaction. Look for an underlying psychological conflict. Another viewpoint is a trait called *alexithymia* (i.e., no words for feelings). This is a psychological style.

Pseudodementia

Also called the dementia of depression. Cognitive symptoms, mainly apathy, concentration difficulty, and refusal to answer, often account for significant memory lapse. Usually the absence of neurological findings, presence of neurovegetative depressive features, acute onset tied to some psychosocial stress, apathy and anhedonia are characteristic of depression and absent in dementias. Normal imaging adds to the presumptive diagnosis of depression.

May be a comorbid early manifestation of a dementia. May also be a manifestation of a psychotic depression (poor concentration, ambivalence, apathy, psychomotor retardation, delusions of poverty or nihilism)

Excess Disability

Often patients with underlying dementia or medical illness have exaggerated disability due to concomitant depression. Function partially improves upon treatment of depression.

Usually a manifestation of a severe depression coexisting with a medical illness.

Psychotic depression in the elderly usually consists of non-bizarre, mood-congruent delusions—for example, a millionaire believing he is bankrupt (delusion of poverty), a patient giving up on treatment because he or she believes nothing will help (nihilistic delusion), refusing help from children because a patient feels he is too much of a burden (delusion of guilt), or being convinced of a terminal illness (somatic delusion). These symptoms are more common than feeling guilty about past deeds or having paranoid delusions. Refusal to eat may be due to a somatic delusion, such as a patient believing that he will explode because he is too thin to fit food inside, or because his constipation means he is blocked up. Psychotic symptoms in older adults can often go unrecognized because, unlike schizophrenia, for example, they are not "bizarre."

Treatment Methods

Medications

Two major sources of information for evidence-based practice are the Agency for Health Care and Quality Research (AHRQ), a branch of the U.S. Department of Health and Human Services, and the Cochrane Collaboration. AHRQ was initially called Agency for Health Care Policy and Research; its new name reflects the fact that it does not determine federal health-care policies. These databases evaluate the quality of studies to facilitate the best medication and treatment selections.

Antidepressants are generally classified by mechanism of action or chemical structure. Medications are classed as selective serotonin reuptake inhibitors (SSRIs), serotonin and norepinephrine reuptake inhibitors (SNRIs), serotonin-2 antagonist reuptake inhibitors (SARIs), noradrenergic specific serotonergic antidepressants (NaSSAs), norepinephrine–dopamine reuptake inhibitors (NDRIs), monoamine oxidase inhibitors (MAOIs), and tricyclic antidepressants (TCAs).

Medications that target the HPA axis, which integrates endocrine, autonomic, and behavioral responses (mood), may be the next point of modulation for depression. Intracellular, mitochondrial receptors have been identified that CRF and other neuropeptides use to control cellular function in depression.

Because these medications interact with other neurotransmitter systems, augmentation for partial responders is suggested for residual symptoms (such as anergy, anxiety, and sleep disturbance) that persist after improvement of depression. An intermediate benzodiazepine such as lorazepam, at 0.5–2 mg/day three or fewer times per week, is allowed as a rescue medication for anxiety during dose titration in most geriatric depression studies and is reasonable in practice. However, clonazepam (Klonopin) and other long-acting benzodiazepines with active metabolites (e.g., diazepam or chlordiazepoxide) are usually avoided in older adults due to the increased risk of "overshooting" (giving too high a dose), accumulation (side effects get worse as time passes), sedation, and unsteady gait that take days to a week to resolve after the medication is discontinued. If sedative antidepressants are insufficient to restore sleep, traditional hypnotics are preferred over other benzodiazepines, trazadone, or diphenhydramine, due to speed of onset.

Several treatment algorithms that follow geriatric prescribing principles of sequential single medication trials, with augmentation for partial responders later in the course of treatment, have been published. The Duke Somatic Treatment Algorithm for Geriatric Depression involves the following stages (Steffans, McQuoid, & Krishnan, 2002):

Stage 1: Start with an SSRI for 6–12 weeks (sertraline).
Stage 2: If there is no response, switch to a previously successful antidepressant for 6–12 weeks. This is usually a TCA but can be another SSRI or other class of antidepressant. If there is only a partial response, augment with bupropion. If there is a full response, maintain the initial SSRI.
Stage 3: If there is no response, switch to venlafaxine for 6–12 weeks. If there is only a partial response, augment with lithium. If there is a full response, maintain the effective medication at the effective dose.
Stage 4: If there is no response, try an SSRI plus TCA (nortriptyline), MAOI, or ECT. If there is a full response, continue venlafaxine and lithium at the effective dose.

Two other well known depression treatment algorithms exist for adult depression but are not specific for elderly: the Texas Medication Algorithm Project (TMAP; Texas Department of State Health Services, 2006) and the NIMH Sequenced Treatment Alternatives to Relieve Depression (STAR-D) study (Travedi et al., 2006; Insel, 2006). They are similar to the staged approach, starting with an SSRI and switching to an NSRI or

TCA as second-line medications. MAOIs are usually tried late in the algorithm. A time-released patch of selegiline (Ensam) seems specific for brain MAOI, and at under 6 mg/day does not cause significant blood pressure problems or dietary precautions, but it has not been studied specifically in older adults.

None of the algorithms specifies optimal doses, but it is widely accepted that many elderly people tend to respond to lower doses of medication, probably due to pharmacokinetic differences, and may benefit at 50% of the average dose for younger adults. The Interpretive Guidelines prepared for OBRA '87 reviewers (Omnibus Budget Reconciliation Act of 1987, which contains nursing home reform regulations) specify a dose range that corresponds with the recommended doses published in the PDR. Generally start at one-half the usual starting dose of a medication and change no more frequently than five half-life intervals (when steady state is achieved) in order to avoid accumulation effects and delayed toxicity from a medication. Note that antipsychotic medication in addition to antidepressants is required to treat psychotic depression. Table 5.3 lists the FDA-approved dose ranges for antipressants by class.

Table 5.3. FDA-Approved Dose Ranges for Antidepressants by Class

CHEMICAL CLASS	GENERIC NAME	TRADE NAME(S)	APPROVED DOSE RANGE (not age specific)
SSRI (selective serotonin reuptake inhibitor)			
Monocyclic	Fluvoxamine	Luvox	50–300 mg/day
Bicyclic	Fluoxetine	Prozac	10–80 mg/day
Phenylpiperidine	Paroxetine	Paxil	20–60 mg/day
	Paroxetine	Paxil CR	12.5–70 mg/day
Phthalane derivatives	Citalopram	Celexa	20–40 mg/day
	Escitalopram	Lexapro	10–20 mg/day
Other	Sertraline	Zoloft	25–200 mg/day
SNRI (serotonin–norepinephrine reuptake inhibitor)	Venlafaxine	Effexor	25–375 mg/day
		Effexor XR	37.5–225 mg/day
	Duloxetine	Cymbalta	20–60 mg/day
		Symbyax (olanzepine with fluoxetine)	6/25–18/75 mg/day

Table 5.3. (continued)

SARI (serotonin-2 antagonist reuptake inhibitor)	Nefazodone Trazodone	Serzone Desyrel	50–600 mg/day 50–600 mg/day
TCA (tricyclic antidepressants = nonselective mixed reuptake inhibitors/ receptor blockers); only secondary TCAs are listed here	Nortriptyline Desipramine	Pamelor Norpramin	10–150 mg/day 10–300 mg/day
NDRI (norepineph-rine–dopamine reuptake inhibitor)	Bupropion	Wellbutrin Wellbutrin-SR, Zyban Wellbutrin-XL	75–400 mg/day (200 bid) 100–400 mg/day 150–450 mg/day
NaSSA (noradrenergic specific serotonergic antidepressant)	Mirtazapine	Remeron	15–45 mg/day
MAOI (monoamine oxidose inhibitor; irreversible) **MAO-A-B** inhibitor	Isocarboxazid Phenelzine Tranylcypromine	Marplan Nardil Parnate	10–60 mg/day 15–90 mg/day 10–60 mg/day

Source: Adapted from Adams (1999).

Electroconvulsive Therapy

Electroconvulsive therapy (ECT) remains the most effective treatment for major depression (American Psychiatric Association, 2001; Rudorfer et al., 1997). The main indications for this treatment are:

- Treatment-resistant mood disorder (at least two adequate medication trials that have failed)
- Psychiatric emergency conditions (e.g., life-threatening anorexia from depression, severe suicide risk, benzodiazepine-resistant catatonia)
- Treatment-resistant mania or schizophrenia

The relative contraindications to this treatment are:

- Severe chronic obstructive pulmonary disease (COPD)
- Severe cardiac disease or recent myocardial infarction
- Severe osteoporosis
- Renal failure (due to hyperkalemia)
- Intracranial neoplasm

There is about an 80% efficacy rate for major depression, and almost all cases are at or close to full remission after an average of six to eight treatments. Treatments are elective and require an informed consent. There is an increasing trend toward outpatient ECT rather than hospitalization.

The mechanism of action, based on experimental epilepsy studies, is induction of biogenic amines, neuropeptides, brain-derived neurotrophic factor (BDNF), and other proteins. Immediate early genes are activated that lead to protein production and ultimately even modification of receptor density and responsiveness (Bazan, 1990). In experimental epilepsy models in rats, the procedure causes neuronal damage if there is hypoxia or status epilepticus leading to glutamate neurotoxicity (an excitatory amino acid).

For the past 50 years, the procedure has been done under anesthesia, and for at least the last 15 years it is usually done in recovery rooms of general hospitals for safety. There is continuous monitoring of oxygen saturation, vital signs, and EEG, with airway management and IV access for medications. Hypertension and tachycardia are the most common side effects and are easily managed with β-blockers. Postictal confusion can occur but is minimized by stimulating the nondominant hemisphere and spacing the interval between treatments. The elderly seems to be the group with the highest rate of ECT use because of intolerance to medication and relative safety of this procedure.

After an ECT series, antidepressant medication must be maintained to reduce the risk of relapse. Without any follow-up, there is about a 50% relapse rate within 6 months.

CASE EXAMPLE

Mrs. C is an 84-year-old woman who had her first depressive episode at age 69. She denies feeling depressed but claims her lips feel numb and her mouth hurts so badly that she stops eating. There is no evidence of oral or neurological pathology. She has no diabetes, hypertension, or major illnesses. Accompanying symptoms are weight loss, constipation, weakness, being bedbound, decreased socialization, difficulty concentrating, psychomotor retardation, and fear of being alone. She says she enjoys visits from her family but does not interact because she feels so badly. Her voice becomes weak and whining. She had a history of depression with classic depressive features when younger, which was effectively treated by imipramine. She noted a recurrence of symptoms when imipramine was discontinued because she started to develop orthostatic hypotension and confusion and intolerance to the medication as she became frailer. Desipramine was ineffective, as were SSRIs. She now requires maintenance with an SNRI and ECT every 4 weeks. She denies any source of worry other than her health. Recently, mild memory deficits have appeared, but attempts to discontinue ECT lead to recurrent somatic complaints.

Diagnosis: *Recurrent major depression (with atypical features) with mild cognitive impairment.*

Psychosocial Interventions

Psychotherapy is effective with older adults and is considered an essential arm of major depression treatment that should be done concomitantly with medication. Differences in technique and approaches are summarized in Chapter 10.

Because of the strong link between geriatric depression and vascular lesions in the brain, some speculate that a possible preventive measure is to limit vascular risk factors by, for example, the cessation of smoking, decreasing alcohol intake, controlling hypertension and diabetes, reducing obesity, and aggressively managing cardiovascular disease.

The current standard of practice requires combined antidepressants and psychotherapy for major depression. Psychotherapy improves response rates and compliance. Patients should acquire improvement in understanding triggering events, knowledge about depression and medications, better coping and communication skills, and a reestablishment of social networks. Insight into longstanding conflictual issues and a decrease in avoidance or denial are also possible as a means to bring about change.

BIPOLAR DISORDER

Background

Bipolar disorder can appear for the first time in late life, although most bipolar patients who are elderly had their first manic episode much earlier in life. Risk factors also include a stroke or dementia as an underlying cause for a first manic episode after age 60. Late-life bipolar patients seem to show less frequent manic episodes about 1%, and depressions appear more treatment resistant. Geriatric mania is also associated with more confusion, paranoia, agitation, irritability, and negativity. Late-onset mania is also different in that it is associated with a lower incidence of family history of mood disorders, longer latency between the first depressive episode and first manic episode (14.9–16 years), and higher association with CNS disorders (43%). This pattern raises unique problems in medication treatment; increased neurotoxicity and confusion may result from existing treatment regimens. For example, elderly patients on long-term lithium management often need to change medications due to emergence of severe coarse tremor and confusion, even when blood levels are maintained at levels below 0.5 mEq/l. There does not appear to be a difference in relapse rates by age (VanGerpen et al., 1999).

Neurobiological Explanation

Mood disorders are phenomenologically viewed as subtypes based on symptoms of mania, hypomania, cyclothymia, rapid cycling, mixed state, and depression, with a family history of mania (incipient cases).

Functional imaging studies with PET, SPECT, and fRMI under a variety of conditions (resting, medicated or not, active disease or remission) show conflicting findings on global brain or lateralized functional changes, but show regional or localized changes with reduced blood flow and metabolism in the frontal lobe and basal ganglia. Equivocal or no changes were found in the temporal lobe, parietal lobe, limbic structures (hippocampal formation, amygdala, uncus), or thalamus. Neuroreceptor imaging studies seem to show state-dependent changes in serotonin and dopamine systems, based on the course of the illness (Soares & Mann, 1997; National Institute of Mental Health, 2007).

Because of the efficacy of diverse agents such as lithium, anticonvulsant medications, and atypical antipsychotic medications in controlling the disorder, the focus of attention turned to signaling networks and cellular signaling pathways. There appears to be abnormalities in G protein subunits in bipolar disorder (Gs/cAMP; stimulatory G protein and increases in postreceptor adenylate cyclase activity). There are also particularly high levels of protein kinase C (PKC) in the brain, which regulate synaptic plasticity. BNDF and other neurotrophic factors needed for the survival and function of neurons seems reduced (Manji, et.al., 2003).

These changes suggest action of medications on membrane stabilization and mitochondrial enzyme impairment that may be the focus for new medication (Tadafumi, 2007). Biological differences between early- and the late-onset bipolar disorder or between subtypes have not been elucidated.

Normal versus Abnormal Behavior

Each phase of the illness has characteristic symptoms, as noted in DSM-IV (American Psychiatric Association, 1994). The main criteria for a manic episode are distinct periods of persistently elevated or expansive mood and/or irritability lasting at least a week. Three or more of seven additional symptoms are required, such as grandiosity, feeling rested despite only 3 or so hours of sleep, pressured speech, racing thoughts, distractibility, psychomotor agitation, and excesses. The criteria for a hypomanic episode are shorter duration of symptoms (3–4 days) and milder additional symptoms (less disruptive). The main criteria for a depressive episode are the same as a major depressive episode. The criteria for a mixed state include meeting criteria for a manic episode and a depressive episode nearly every day for at least 1 week.

A longstanding theory of "kindling" holds that the first episode of bipolar disorder is associated with a major psychological stress (i.e., an external stressor) but as neurobiological changes become permanent, whatever they are, further episodes occur without external triggers. This pattern does seem to be present in older adults' inability to identify clear precipitants (Axis IV).

Unique Aspects of the Disorder in Elderly

One aspect that requires special attention is the possibility of secondary mania. Table 5.4 provides a list of diseases and medications associated with manic symptoms.

Table 5.4. Causes of Secondary Mania

NEUROLOGICAL DIESASES	SUBSTANCES
Alzheimer's disease	Alcohol
Parkinson's disease	Benzodiazepines
Pick's disease	Tricyclic antidepressants
Epilepsy	Bronchodilators
Neurosyphillis and encephalopathies	Bupropion
Normal pressure hyrocephalus	Decongestants
Systemic illness	Dexatrim
Hyperthyroidism	Calcium replacement
Other endocrine dysfunctions	Cimetidine
Influenza	Corticosteroids
End-stage renal disease/dialysis	Anabolic steroids

Source: Adapted from VanGerpen et al. (1999).

Assessment and Diagnosis

The process of assessment to rule out the possible causes of secondary mania requires a psychiatric interview with a focus on family history and concomitant drug and alcohol use and medical screening that includes baseline laboratory tests (usually done by internal medicine). The diagnosis, like all forms of psychiatric illness, is still a clinical one. There are no laboratory tests or genetic tests to verify the diagnosis. There is often a family history of bipolar illness or schizophrenia and a relatively high rate of alcohol abuse.

Treatment Methods

Medications
Choices for treating bipolar disorder in older adults are similar to those for younger adults, but options may be limited due to poor tolerance or coexisting disease contraindications. Each phase of bipolar illness—depressed phase, manic phase, maintenance phase

(euthymia)—has different approved medications. Mixed states have not been well studied, and recommendations are generally based on limited data and have a relatively low level of confidence.

Treatment of bipolar illness is one of the few arenas that even geriatric psychiatrists deviate from the single-medication rule. However, combination therapies even for general adult populations, such as recommendations about treatment of mixed states, are generally Class IV data with Level D confidence. Table 5.5 reflects choices based on existing literature, with parenthetical comments reflecting my personal preferences.

Table 5.5. FDA-Approved Medications for Bipolar Disorder Phases

MANIC PHASE
1. All antipsychotics have indications (atypical antipsychotics are typically first line)
2. Lithium
3. Valproate

DEPRESSED PHASE
1. All antidepressants have indications (bupropion, venlafaxine, or SSRIs are first line)
2. Lithium
3. Olanzepine

MAINTENANCE PHASE
1. Lithium
2. Lamotrigine
3. Olanzepine
4. Symblax (fluoxetine and olanzepine)
5. Aripiprizole

MIXED STATES
1. Atypical antipsychotic—e.g., olanzepine
2. Maintain with a maintenance medication; use antidepressants short term during depressive phase

---

Case reports of "effective" combination therapies in general adult patients include:

- Lithium with valproate
- Lithium with carbamazepine
- Lithium with calcium channel blockers
- Lithium with lamotrigine

- Lithium with clozapine
- Lithium with novel antipsychotics (e.g., risperidone, olanzapine)
- Valproate with antipsychotics
- Valproate with lamotrigine

Warnings:

- Lithium with traditional antipsychotics may have increased neurotoxicity (a black-box warning in the PDR).
- Metabolic syndrome is a warning for all novel antipsychotics (ziprasidone and aripiprazole may cause the least risk).
- Lithium often leads to the emergence of a coarse tremor, cognitive impairment, and rising creatinine in older adults at previously therapeutic blood levels. Often therapeutic levels for lithium in the elderly are as low as 0.3 mEq/l. If side effects do not improve after dose reduction, the medication must be stopped.
- Many elderly patients on chronic lithium need levothyroxine (Synthroid) without development of goiter. It is unclear if this is a lithium side effect.

Even in older adults, lithium is generally the medication of choice for maintenance unless there is renal insufficiency or significant confusion. Divalproate has traditionally been the second choice and carbamazepine the third. Time-release forms of lithium may improve compliance and reduce adverse effects by eliminating peaks and troughs in blood levels. Combination medication for maintenance has become the norm in younger patients. To repeat: This is one exception to the general rule of using a medication with an indication first.

SUICIDE

Background

Rates as high as 50/100,000 are seen in older white men compared to baseline rates of about 10/100,000 for suicide in the general population. Seventy-five percent of completed suicides are by firearms, although frail elderly are also more likely to succumb to less invasive means of suicide, such as overdoses. If one counts starvation from depression as indirect suicide, then the suicide rates are even higher. Additional information about suicide in late life is available from Established Populations for Epidemiologic Studies of the Elderly (EPESE; Turvey et al., 2002).

The basic assumption is that suicide follows a trajectory that starts with risk factors leading to death wishes, which progress to suicidal ideation, and culminate in a suicide attempt. This course implies that there are early warning signs.

The main premorbid risks of suicide are depression, substance abuse, chronic disability, catastrophic loss, or strong genetic or experiential loading (e.g., a family member committed suicide). These factors may lead to a death wish expressed by patients as "I wish God would take me" or "I wish something would happen to me so I would die." Lack of improvement or addition of new losses or failures lead to suicidal ideation to end the suffering. The final act is hard to predict because it is, by and large, impulsive. Many patients have suicidal thoughts for many years. What would lead such an individual with chronic suicidal ideation to finally make a suicide attempt? Inherently, the cause is "one last straw that broke the camel's back." This is why it is so important to try to remove stressors and increase social support (buffers) when a patient is suicidal. This pattern is shown graphically in Figure 5.1.

Figure 5.1. Risk factors, precipitants, and buffers of suicide in older adults.

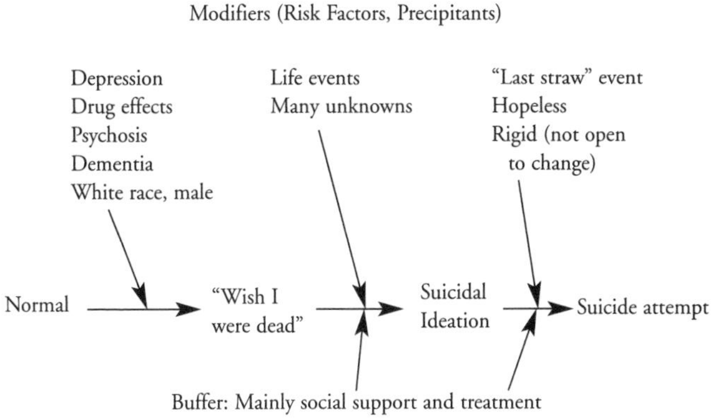

Modifiers (Risk Factors, Precipitants)

Depression   Life events   "Last straw" event
Drug effects   Many unknowns   Hopeless
Psychosis   Rigid (not open
Dementia   to change)
White race, male

Normal → "Wish I were dead" → Suicidal Ideation → Suicide attempt

Buffer: Mainly social support and treatment

Factors that increase impulsive acts, such as substance abuse, psychosis (e.g., command hallucinations), or dementia with suicidal ideation are less predictable and require closer supervision.

Unique Aspects of the Disorder in Elderly

Depression is the most common cause of suicide in older patients. Unlike younger patients, schizophrenia or substance abuse is not as commonly associated, but pain and sleep deprivation are.

Assessment and Diagnosis

Prediction of imminent risk is the major task of an evaluation. Hospitalization is needed for protection of the patient with serious suicidal risk. Table 5.6 summarizes levels of risk for suicide in older adults.

Table 5.6. Levels of Risk for Suicide in Older Adults

INCREASED BASELINE RISK
- Depression
- Lives alone
- Widowed
- Lacks confidante
- Elderly white male
- Recent major stress or loss
- Alcoholism
- Prior suicide attempt
- Family history of suicide

INCREASED IMMEDIATE RISK (NEED FOR HOSPITALIZATION)
- Hopelessness (not open to new experience; can't see "light at the end of the tunnel")
- Highly lethal plan (e.g., gun)
- Suicidal thoughts, plus—
  - Psychosis
  - Cognitive impairment
  - Panic attacks
  - Agitation
  - Incapacitating anxiety
  - Moderate alcohol abuse
- Suicidal thoughts, without—
  - Social support
  - Therapeutic relationship
- Global insomnia (panic about not getting to sleep)

Table 5.6. (continued)

OUTPATIENT CARE USUALLY POSSIBLE IF ALL OF THE FOLLOWING
ARE PRESENT
- Attempt is a reaction to a precipitating event, often with secondary gain (impulsive)
- Plan/method and intent have low lethality
- Stable and supportive living situation
- Able to cooperate with follow-up
- Has chronic suicidal ideation without intent
- Overdose was accidental (e.g., for pain control)

Source: Based on McCrae & Costa (1990) and American Psychiatric Association (2003).

Having a plan for suicide is not always a sign of imminent action, but it is important to safety proof the patient's environment to prevent ease of action (e.g., take away guns or means of suicide). A more important predictor of a suicidal act is a patient's sense of hopelessness and rigidity (i.e., not being open to change; McCrae & Costa, 1990). Other imminent risks are global insomnia, severe anxiety with panic attacks, psychosis, or substance abuse (because intoxication increases impulsivity and unpredictability; Busch & Fawcett, 2004; American Psychiatric Association, 2004).

Treatment Methods

Medications
Medication for the primary diagnosis is needed. There is no guidance about which medications may be differentially more or less effective for suicidal ideation. The FDA held hearings about extending the warning to adults about increased risk of suicidality (suicidal thinking and behavior) in children and adolescents treated with SSRIs, but found insufficient data to do so. The actual warning in the PDR also stated "Anyone considering the use of an antidepressant in a child or adolescent for any clinical use must balance the risk of increased suicidality with the clinical need" (FDA, 2007).

Psychosocial Interventions
Treatment of the underlying source of stress and removing risk factors such as depression or substance abuse are an essential part

of suicide intervention. Patients with chronic suicidal ideation can usually be treated on an outpatient basis if a therapeutic alliance has been established and the following conditions exist:

- Possibility of frequent sessions (transportation, affordability, availability of MD)
- Availability of social supports for the patient (lives with someone or someone can stay in the home)
- Mobilization of outpatient care.

Making a therapeutic contract with the patient to call before making a suicide attempt and accept hospitalization is possible if the patient is ambivalent (a part of him or her wants to live), is cognitively intact, is not psychotic, and has a strong therapeutic alliance with the doctor. Hospitalization is needed when suicidal intent is high or the patient is impulsive, such as a suicidal patient with a history of impulsive acts, cognitive impairment, psychosis, or active substance abuse.

CASE EXAMPLE

The following case exemplifies points made in the chapter about the differential diagnosis of depression in late life and medication prescribing issues.

Presenting Complaint
I just don't have the energy that I used to. Is something wrong with me?

History
Mrs. J is an 82-year-old woman with no siblings, whose husband died 4 years ago. She married at age 23 and they were happily married for 55 years. She said she and her husband were insepa-rable. The patient said their 60th anniversary was coming up and she still keeps his clothes in the closet. She initially thought she saw her husband in the room after his death. Mrs. J. is a college graduate and a retired kindergarten teacher. Her four adult chil-dren are married and live out-of-state. She denies depression but has no pleasure in what she does anymore. She is still socially

active, but has to force herself to go out. She complains of anergy, low back pain, has difficulty staying asleep, believes her sense of taste has changed since no food tastes good anymore, but denies a change in weight. She has been on lorazepam for chronic anxiety for 4 years now at a stable dose. There is no gross psychomotor retardation, and no suicidal ideation or death wishes. Medical evaluation revealed normal thyroid function and no cardiac, renal, or other medical problems.

The patient's father died of a heart attack when she was 12. Her mother, who was 35 when he died, never remarried. The patient believes her life changed markedly afterward due to financial hardship and her mother's depression. They ultimately moved in with a maternal aunt.

This case represents many common features of late life depression. This was the first major depressive episode for this patient. Hallucinations are seen in almost 50% of widows in the first few weeks after loss. Signs of pathological mourning include "mummification" of the house (will not change anything), continuing to observe anniversaries as if the deceased is still alive, and dysthymia or depression. The sensitizing effect of her parent loss as a pre-teen and the biological predisposition of depression in her mother are significant risk factors for the patient's depression. Her small family size and lack of nearby relatives add to the risk for depression.

The patient responded well to an SSRI and psychotherapy. She was guided through appropriate mourning with Interpersonal Psychotherapy (ITP). Augmentation or medication changes were not needed in this case, but are often needed due to higher rates of adverse effects in the elderly, or less robust effects in initial treatments. Use of an antipsychotic was not required despite her reports of hallucinations because they were episodic and not disruptive.

SUMMARY

Mood disorders are very common psychiatric disorders among the elderly, and depression is the most common, almost always occurring with anxiety. Compared to younger patients, the main differences in late life depression are vascular depression and the presence of medical causes behind the depressive symptoms. The choice of medication is the same as general adult depression treatment algorithms, but lower doses are usually required. ECT is the treatment of choice for treatment-resistant depression or psychiatric emergencies such as severe suicidality. Psychosocial interventions are also important. In addition to depression, late-onset bipolar illness can occur in the elderly. Treatment of bipolar disorder in the elderly is different than in younger adults due to higher rates of adverse events that preclude the use of many medications. Lithium is often poorly tolerated, leading to the more frequent use of depakote or novel antipsychotics for maintenance in bipolar disease.

6

PSYCHOSIS

Psychosis in late life is usually divided into early-onset and late-onset forms. Early-onset psychotic disorders are usually due to schizophrenia or bipolar disorders. Late-onset psychosis is mainly related to major depression, dementia, and delirium (Webster & Grossberg, 1998), as noted in Table 6.1. Late-onset schizophrenia, labeled *paraphrenia* by Emil Kraeplin in the 19th century, refers to a disorder similar to paranoid schizophrenia, but with late onset and less personality deterioration. Kraeplin initially viewed paraphrenia as a form of insanity related to transitional periods of life (adolescent and senile forms) because it seemed to have a different presentation and course than typical schizophrenia. Paraphrenia is labeled an atypical psychosis or delusional disorder (American Psychiatric Association, 2000).

Table 6.1. Admissions for Psychosis in Older Adults

Dementia (40%)
Psychotic depression (33%)
Delirium (11%)
Medical related (7%)
Bipolar disorder (2%)
Delusional disorder (2%)
Not well characterized (2%)
Schizophrenia (2%)
Schizoaffective disorder (1%)

Source: Based on Webster & Grossberg (1998).

BACKGROUND

The difference in the presentation of older psychotic patients suggests different pathophysiology for paraphrenia, psychotic depression, and psychosis associated with AD.

Neurobiological Explanation

Psychosis involves changes in the dopaminergic, cholinergic, and serotonergic systems, which are further modulated by the excitatory (glutamate) and inhibitory (GABA) systems. The differences in presentation and associated disorders may reflect different abnormalities in the various systems. It is speculated that psychotic symptoms in younger adults with schizophrenia involve excess dopamine activity in the mesolimbic area, psychotic depression with decreased activity in the serotonergic system, and psychosis in dementia with decreased cholinergic activity. Acetycholine and serotonin both modulate the dopamine system.

Historically, serotonin (5-HT, 5-hydroxytryptophan) was thought to cause psychosis because LSD induced its effect by blocking 5-HT from binding to its receptor. The presence of 5-HT seems to prevent the release of dopamine, and suppressed serotonin function, as occurs in depression, increases dopamine release and, in severe depression, leads to psychosis.

As a brief review (see Davis et al., 2002), the dopamine family of receptors (D_n) is divided into two discrete classes, the D_1-like family (D_1 and D_5/D_{1B}) and the D_2-like family (D_2, D_3, D_4). Each receptor type is distributed in different areas of the brain and projects to different brain areas. Generally the D_2-like family of receptors cluster in the mesolimbic system and lead to psychotic symptoms when dopamine activity is high. A decrease in D_2-like family receptor agonists in the nigrostriatal pathway leads to extrapyramidal symptoms. Decreased agonism of D_1-like family receptors, clustered in the frontal lobe, is thought to cause negative symptoms.

5-HT receptors are divided into seven discrete families, each with different clustering in the brain and different projections. The 5-HT_1 family (1A, 1B, 1C, 1D, 1E), 5-HT_2 family (2A, 2B,

2C, 3, 4), and 5-HT$_5$ family seem to have psychiatric relevance. 5-HT neurons project to dopaminergic pathways in several areas: the caudate nucleus, putamen, nucleus accumbens, amygdala, and medial prefrontal cortex. The 5-HT$_1$ family seems to inhibit dopamine system function. The low serotonin function in depression (inferred from lower cerebrospinal fluid 5-HT levels), coupled with low acetylcholinergic function may account for the seemingly higher rate of psychosis associated with major depression in older adults, as well as mood disturbance in psychotic disorders.

NMDA receptor-mediated glutamate transmission is also implicated in psychosis (Harrison & Weinberger, 2005). Glutamate, an excitatory neurotransmitter, interacts closely with dopamine and serotonin systems, and prolonged NMDA–glutamate receptor antagonism or heightened glutamate activity is known to cause psychotic symptoms, as with phencyclidine (phenyl cyclohexyl piperidine [PCP]). There are also direct and indirect links between serotonin, dopamine, and GABA signaling.

Cholinergic dysfunction has also been implicated as a cause of psychosis (Cummings & Back, 1998). Atrophy of the nucleus basalis of Meynert, the principle site of acetylcholine manufacture, are known to occur in AD, and these cholinergic neurons project to the limbic system and neocortex. Both the cholinergic and glutamatergic causes of psychosis contribute to the transient symptomatology seen in those psychoses that are associated with AD.

Finding genetic associations for these putative causes for psychosis has proven elusive. There is not one gene for one enzyme, as was originally thought. The same gene sequence produces different messenger ribonucleic acid (mRNA) and proteins based on other promoter genes, and the environmental factors that lead to gene expression or inhibition are appearing to be increasingly complicated. There have been no pedigrees to study whereby one could observe genetically simple Mendelian inheritance (Kendler, 2006). There will be strong treatment implications for psychosis if the cellular, genetic, and molecular characterization of a core molecular pathway and a "genetic cytoarchitecture" (Harrison & Weinberger, 2005) are elucidated.

Normal Versus Abnormal Behavior

Despite the heterogeneity in putative causes, psychosis is still characterized symptomatically along the positive and negative symptom scale originally described for schizophrenia (Kay et al., 1987). Even for schizophrenia, controversy existed as to whether there were just two distinct dimensions to a formal thought disorder, or more. The current definition of psychosis usually emphasizes positive symptoms to make the diagnosis. Negative symptoms and other aspects of thought disorders—such as somatic concern, anxiety, guilt, tension, abnormal mannerisms, depression, psychomotor retardation, uncooperativeness, unusual thought content, disorientation, poor attention, judgment and insight, disturbance of volition, poor impulse control, preoccupations and social avoidance—vary. Positive symptoms (putatively related to D_2 receptor stimulation in the mesolimbic system) include:

- Delusions
- Conceptual disorganization (e.g., paralogical, circumstantial)
- Hallucinatory behavior
- Excitement
- Grandiosity
- Suspiciousness or persecutory ideation
- Hostility

Negative symptoms (putatively related to reduced D_1 receptor stimulation in the frontal cortex and subcortical abnormality) include:

- Blunted affect
- Emotional withdrawal
- Poor rapport
- Passive or apathetic, socially withdrawn
- Impaired abstract thinking
- Lack of spontaneity
- Stereotyped thinking and difficulty changing topics

Symptomatic differences between schizophrenia, paraphrenia, and psychosis in Alzheimer's disease (AD) are listed in Table 6.2.

Table 6.2. Symptomatic Differences between Schizophrenia, Paraphrenia, and Psychosis in AD

SCHIZOPHRENIA	PARAPHRENIA	PSYCHOSIS IN AD
Complex delusions	Paranoid delusions	Simple delusions
Auditory hallucinations (visual hallucinations are rare)	Auditory hallucinations (visual hallucinations are rare)	Visual and auditory hallucinations
Suicidal ideation common	Premorbid schizoid tendencies	Suicidal ideation rare
Remission of psychosis rare	Deafness common	Remission of psychosis (even in same day) common
Caregiver misidentification rare	Caregiver misidentification rare	Caregiver misidentification common
Past history of psychosis common	Past history of psychosis rare, but positive family history	Past history of psychosis rare
Negative symptoms common	Less negative symptoms or "deterioration"	Apathy common, other negative symptoms less so

Source: Based on Jeste & Finkel (2000); Jeste et al. (2004); Deutsch et al. (1991); Cummings et al. (1994).

In general, psychotic ideation in older adults is less bizarre and simpler than delusions in schizophrenia. A simple delusion is an almost believable belief, unless one knows the real social setting, and it does not cause as much impairment. Examples of simple delusions are:

- Belief that others plan to hurt one.
- Belief that others are stealing.
- Belief that the spouse is having an affair.
- Belief that an unwelcome guest is living in the house.
- Belief that the spouse or others are not who they claim to be (delusion of doubles—Capgrass syndrome).
- Belief that one's house is not one's home.
- Belief that family members plan to abandon one.
- Belief that television or magazine figures are present.

- Describes hearing voices or acts as if one does.
- Talks to people who are not there (usually long deceased relatives).
- Describes seeing things not seen by others (people, animals, lights).
- Reports smelling odors not smelled by others.
- Describes feeling things on one's skin.

Unique Aspects of the Disorder in Elderly

Because the delusions are less bizarre than in schizophrenia, it is often easier to see that their content has personal relevance to the patient in explaining unwelcome changes, although the thoughts themselves are false and illogical. This content relevance applies not only to paraphrenia, but to the psychosis of dementia and psychotic depression. That is, the content has meaning to an empathic listener and represents the patient's psychic reality. Often the symptoms can be seen as restitutive, that is, as gratifying some need. For example, a sense of failure and rejection in personal relationships is compensated by persecutory delusions that allow the patient to believe that others are jealous of him or her and that he or she is the center of attention. This viewpoint, discussed in great detail in Arieti's *Interpretation of Schizophrenia* (revised edition in 1994) and *The Course of Life* (Greenspan & Pollock, 1980), offers guidance to what is needed in supportive therapy or social interventions.

The following case is an example of this point. The patient always showed schizoid traits (i.e., a preschizophrenic personality), but did not manifest frank delusions until she developed a sensory impairment and retired from her daily routine of work. The content of her delusions suggests that she is fearful of losing anything more (hoarding) and sensitive to her growing social isolation (becomes the center of attention in her delusion, albeit in a negative way).

CASE EXAMPLE

Mrs. J is an 73-year-old woman who has been characterized as eccentric and shy throughout life. Although she was a college graduate, she never advanced beyond an office pool secretary. She never married and her pastor and family said she was always socially isolative. After retiring from work and becoming hard of hearing, she became a virtual recluse. She began to think people were talking about her behind her back and making fun of her. If people laughed in her presence, she was sure they were laughing at her. She developed persecutory delusions around a neighbor breaking in to steal her things. She moved to escape this perceived possibility, but then became convinced that her new neighbor was following her and was enlisting the help of others in the new apartment building to spy on her and break in if they had the chance. The patient increased her hoarding behavior. A neighbor ultimately reported her to the police because the apartment had become a fire safety hazard from stored papers. The evaluation did not reveal significant cognitive impairment, medical illness, or depression. The patient was not taking any prescribed medications, and denied alcohol use or drugs. She responded well to antipsychotics and supportive psychotherapy, and to having her pastor and old church members visit her. She never gained insight into her illness. She was just thankful that the people had stopped bothering, attributing it to their fear of being "found out" by the doctors who were now involved in her life.

ASSESSMENT AND DIAGNOSIS

Interviewing patients with paranoia or dementia may be difficult because they are usually defensive and offer little spontaneous information. Collateral information is often needed to elaborate on the patient's behaviors and beliefs and to verify if the content is true or delusional.

For nonverbal patients or those showing severe denial, the use of informants is especially important to ascertain behavior patterns (e.g., nocturnal symptoms only) and provide detail that the patient will not reveal. Patients may often admit to having "dreams" that are actually hallucinations. Differentiation is made by asking if the dreams (1) persist after the patient awakens, (2) last longer than hypnopompic hallucinations (dream-like hallucinations as one wakes up) that might be seen in a primary sleep disorder, (3) seem to occur outside of their head (i.e., not just a preoccupation or thought), or (4) occur during the day.

Psychosis in patients with AD often tends to occur episodically at night, and patients usually do not recall the event. In nursing homes, patients often do not show any psychotic ideation when evaluated, but staff lament, "The patient always acts nicely when you come." The real problems occur at night when patients report hearing someone screaming and are afraid that someone is being killed or that intruders are lurking. This diurnal variation is not typical of paraphrenia or schizophrenia.

As mentioned in earlier chapters, delirium, medication side effects, and illnesses such as thyroid disease should always be a major consideration as a cause for an acute psychotic episode or exacerbation. Additional diagnostic testing should be done to rule out medical instability. If warranted by the history, toxicology, heavy metal screening, syphilis, hepatitis C, and HIV testing should be done. Baseline physical and laboratory assessments and a physical examination should be conducted before starting an antipsychotic, because a baseline is needed to compare for possible emergent adverse effects (American Psychiatric Association, 2004). An initial assessment should be made for Parkinson symptoms and preexisting obesity and diabetes, which may be worsened with antipsychotic medications. The recommended frequency of monitoring is discussed in Chapter 2 and suggests quarterly checkups initially, with at least annual checks on the following:

- Vital signs (pulse, blood pressure, temperature)
- Body weight and height and note diabetes risk factors
- CBC, electrolytes, renal function tests (BUN/creatinine), liver function tests, thyroid function tests
- Fasting blood sugar (FBS), lipid panel
- Hemoglobin AlC if patient is diabetic
- EKG (especially baseline QTc) and concomitant medications that might prolong QTc
- Extrapyramidal symptom (EPS) evaluation to determine early Parkinson's and risk for falls and tardive dyskinesia (TD) (see Table 6.3)
- Screening for symptoms of hyperprolactinemia, including baseline prolactin levels, may be needed if older antipsychotics are used

TREATMENT METHODS

Medications

Medications for psychosis, irrespective of the cause, still revolve around the addition of an antipsychotic medication. The doses are ideally titrated from low to therapeutic levels (covered in Chapter 2). It is important to continue to titrate a single medication to efficacy or maximum allowed dose before adding another medication to avoid adverse effects.

Target symptoms should also be clear. Improvement in "positive psychotic target symptoms" (thought disorder, delusions, and hallucinations) should be the main indication of improvement rather than reduction of aggression or hyperactivity. Medication doses should be increased slowly until the target symptoms improve; this will often be higher than the dose that brings about initial calming. The target dose is typically based on a consensus of experts rather than studies at this time. Atypical antipsychotics can also cause EPS and TD, although at a much lower rate than traditional antipsychotics. The examination should cover the areas noted in Table 6.3.

Table 6.3. Rating Movement Disorders Using AIMS and EPS

AIMS (Abnormal Involuntary Movement Scale for Tardive Dyskinesia)
    Facial and oral movements
    Extremity movements (upper and lower)
    Trunk movements (neck, shoulders, hip—rocking, twisting, gyrating, grunting)
    Patient's awareness of movements and degree of incapacity

EPS (Extrapyramidal Symptoms)
    Gait (stance, propulsion, arm swing, turning)
    Rigidity
        —Arm dropping (hold arms at shoulder height and let them fall)
        —Shoulder shaking (rotate humerus) to check for rigidity
        —Elbow rigidity (extend and flex at the elbow)
        —Wrist rigidity
        —Head (move head from side to side)
    Glabella tap
    Tremor (observe with arms held out and fingers spread)
    Salivation
    Akathisia

Table 6.3. (continued)

It is usually helpful to induce subtle movements through activation (e.g., ask the patient to extend arms or stick out tongue) or to distract the patient from conscious attempts at reducing movements (e.g., ask the patient to tap thumb on finger while observing other parts of body).

Although these areas can be scored, it is usually sufficient to note any abnormalities as a chart note.

Source: Based on Munetz & Benjamin (1988; AIMS); and Simpson & Angus (1970; EPS).

Because EPS are associated with falls and later development of TD, if EPS occurs, the first step is to reduce the dose of medication. If adverse effects continue, change to a different novel antipsychotic medication.

Treatment of medication-induced akathisia is usually addressed by dose reduction or change rather than adding β-blockers or other medications.

Emergence of TD is treated by discontinuation of the antipsychotic. If a medication-free period cannot be managed, switch to a different novel antipsychotic medication.

For older adults who have a major depressive disorder with psychotic features, a combination of SSRI or SNRI and a novel antipsychotic is needed. Each disorder, depression and psychosis, requires individual dose titrations to efficacy for both symptom components.

Antipsychotic response seems to be quite rapid in older adults with dementia and psychosis. Even a single, low, nightly dose with a short-acting antipsychotic can suppress psychotic symptoms for the entire day, with effects seen within days of starting the medication.

There are no age-specific evidence-based treatment algorithms for the elderly population. The NIMH CATIE study did head-to-head comparisons of antipsychotics for both schizophrenia (Lieberman et al., 2005) and psychosis associated with AD (Schneider et al., 2006). In the CATIE schizophrenia trial, 227 patients were randomized into:

• First-generation medication (chlorpromazine, droperidol, flupenthixol, flupenthixol decaonoate, fluphenazine decanoate,

haloperidol, haloperidol decanoate, loxapine, methotrimeprazine, pepotiazine palmitate, sulpiride, thioridazine, trifluoperazine hydrochloride, zuclopenthixol, and zuclopenthixol decanoate), *versus*
- A second-generation medication (amilsulpride, olanzapine, quetiapine, risperidone).
- If there was poor tolerance or no effect by week 12, the medication was switched.
- If there was improvement, the same medication was continued for up to 52 weeks.

The CATIE AD trial randomized patients into:

- Second-generation antipsychotics only (olanzapine, quetiapine, and risperidone) because of higher adverse effects with first-generation medications.
- If there was poor tolerance or no effect by week 12, the medication was switched.

This AD protocol is similar to guidelines from the American Psychiatric Association (2004) and Texas Medication Algorithm Project (Texas Department of State Health Services 2003), which start with atypical antipsychotics. Protocols begin to deviate lower in the algorithm. Some continue to switch to single new medication, others switch to clozaril, others begin to augment with a second antipsychotic. The general geriatric prescribing principles still apply, however. Switching between sequential single medication trials is preferable to polypharmacy, and it is preferable to start at 50% the usual starting dose, increase rapidly to the target dose based on geriatric studies (usually 50% of the average adult dose), and then continue to advance slowly (at five half-life intervals) until target symptoms begin to improve or the maximum recommended dose is reached.

If a partial response occurs, augmentation may be considered. If the patient has plateaued on maximum doses of a novel antipsychotic, a clinician can give a small dose of a nonsedative first-generation antipsychotic, such as low-dose haloperidol (Haldol) or perphenazine (Trilafon), to increase D_2 receptor blockade above what is possible with a novel antipsychotic. The older norm was that 60–80% D_2 receptor blocade is needed for an antipsychotic response in schizophrenia. Clozapine (Clozaril) is still considered late or last in the treatment algorithm for older adults. It requires WBC monitoring.

In terms of efficacy, there were no significant differences between first- and second-generation antipsychotics in the CATIE trials. However, quality-of-life measures, such as functional status and life satisfaction, tended to be greater for the second-generation medications (Jones et al., 2006).

Atypical antipsychotics are preferred for long-term use with older adults because of lower rates of TD (5% for second-generation antipsychotics as opposed to 20% incidence rate for first-generation antipsychotics; Jeste et al., 2000). Even for short-term use, older (first-generation) antipsychotics cause significantly more confusion and EPS at therapeutic doses.

Unlike treatment for schizophrenia, the use of benzodiazepines is usually not recommended as concomitant treatment due to the possibility of resulting confusion and falls. In intensive care units, lorazepam has been found to be an independent risk factor for transitioning to delirium (Pandharipande et al., 2006). If needed for agitation, benzodiazepines are usually restricted for the acute phase of illness, but should be discontinued in the stabilization phase, and the lowest possible dose should be used to avoid side effects. Lorazepam is usually given at doses of 0.5–1 mg per day (divided doses).

Maintenance with antipsychotics is recommended in psychotic disorders for periods exceeding 6 months. Even when stable and not needing psychotherapy, patients should be seen two to four times per year as long as they are on medication. Lifetime maintenance on medications is advisable for patients who have had recurrent psychotic episodes after prior medication discontinuations. Although there is no evidence for it, most clinicians taper medications slowly (over 2 weeks) rather than stopping medications.

Table 6.4 is a slight modification of Table 4.6 with a broader range of antipsychotics listed, available doses, and cytochrome P450 enzyme profiles that predict medication interactions.

Table 6.4. Antipsychotic Recommendations for Geriatric Patients

MEDICATION	STARTING DOSE TARGET DOSE (approved range in PDR)	COMMENTS

Aripiprazole	Start 2 mg/day
	Target 10 mg/day
	(2–30 mg/day)
		2, 5, 10, 15, 20,
		  30 mg and solution
		Long half-life—
		  steady state takes 2 weeks
		CYP2D6 inhibitors such as
		  fluoxetine and paroxetine
		  require 50% dose
		  reduction
		CYP2D6 inducers such as
		  carbamazepine require
		  50% dose increase

Olanzapine (Zyprexa,
  Zydis Zyprexa IM)
	Start 2.5–5 mg/day
	Target 10 mg/day
	(2.5–20 mg/day)
		2.5, 5, 7.5, 10, 15,
		  20 mg tablet;
		5, 10, 15, 20 mg
		  disintegrating; 10 mg
		  injection

Risperidone (Risperdal,
  Consta, M-tab)
	Start 0.25 mg/day
	Dementia 0.75–1.5 mg/day
	(0.25–16 mg/day oral)
		0.25, 0.5, 1, 2, 3,
		  4 mg tablet;
		0.5, 1, 2 mg disintegrating;
		  1 mg/ml solution and
		  25, 37.5, 50 mg IM

Paliperidone (Invega)	Start 3 mg qd (no data on elderly)	3, 6, 9 mg tablet
Quetiapine (Seroquel)	Start 25 mg qd or bid Target 100–200 mg/day (25–800 mg/day)	25, 100, 200, 300 mg tablet

Ziprasidone (Geodon)	Start 20 mg qd or bid
	Target 20–40 mg bid
	(20–80 mg bid oral)
		20, 40, 60, 80 mg and
		  short-acting IM
		  (mesylate form)
		More effect on QTc
		50% increase in absorption
		  with food

Haloperidol (Haldol)	Start 0.5 mg/day
	Target 2–5 mg/day
	(up to 100 mg/day [oral]
	has been used in resistant
	patients)
		0.5, 1, 2, 5, 10, 20 mg
		  scored tablet; 2 mg/ml
		  solution and both short-
		  acting and long-acting
		  (decanoate form)

Table 6.4. (continued)

MEDICATION	STARTING DOSE TARGET DOSE (approved range in PDR)	COMMENTS
		IV haloperidol, used in ICU settings, increases QTc and has had reports of Torsade de Pointes
Perphenazine (Trilafon)	Start 2 mg/day Target 4–8 mg (max 64 mg/day)	2, 4, 8, 16 mg tablet
Fluphenazine (Prolixin)	Start 1 mg/day Target 1–2 mg/day (max 40 mg/day)	1, 5, 10 mg tablet; also elixir and long-acting IM (decanoate form)
Colazapine (Clozaril)	Start 12.5 mg qd Target 100 mg/day Parkinson's 25 mg/day (max 900 mg/day)	12.5, 25, 100 mg tablet; risk of agranolocytosis and seizures. WBC monitor ing weekly for 6 months, every 2 weeks for the next 6 months, and at least every 4 weeks until 1 month after discontin uation

NO LONGER ADVISED FOR ELDERLY

Chlorpromazine (Thorazine)		Causes orthostatic hypotension and confusion
Thioridazine (Mellaril)		Causes orthostatic hypotension and confusion
Diphenhydramine (Benadryl)		Although not an antipsy chotic, it is frequently prescribed for sleep or EPS (if first-generation antipsychotics are used), but should not be prescribed

Cognitive impairment related to the disorganization from psychosis, considered a "negative symptom of schizophrenia," is usually not treated with medication, but trials have been done with glutamatergic agents and AChEIs in patients with schizophrenia, with mild benefits (American Psychiatric Association, 2004).

ECT remains the major alternative for treatment-resistant psychosis as well as treatment-resistant depression and catatonia (when benzodiazepines fail).

Psychosocial Interventions

Applying the biopsychosocial model is important. Using the formula "Predisposition + Precipitant + Perpetuating Circumstances = Negative Outcome," successful treatment should incorporate an intervention for every contributing factor, as summarized in Table 6.5.

Table 6.5. Contributing Factors Requiring Treatment in the Biopsychosocial Model

PROBLEM CATEGORY	EXAMPLES	TREATMENT
Predispositions	Genetic loading Early life experience Financial worries	Long-term antipsychotic use Psychotherapy Social work services
Precipitant	Trauma Death of a loved one Financial loss Interpersonal conflict	Social services Psychotherapy Social skill building (nondemented), supportive care, and tolerance (demented)
Perpetuating circumstances	Ongoing interpersonal conflicts or the reverse of social isolation Poverty Housing problem Poor social skills	Cognitive–behavioral therapy (coping skills, problem solving) Family interventions (restore support network, educate family about medications and course) Social services (financial planning) Housing (with supports)
Outcome (psychosis)	Symptomatic treatment	Mainly antipsychotic use

The psychological approaches for psychosis can be divided into an acute phase, stabilization phase, and maintenance phase.

In the acute phase, psychosocial interventions involve reducing stimulation, improving conflictual relationships, and reducing environmental stress. A structured and predictable setting must be created that is tolerant of deviance (not just tolerant of aggression) and has low performance expectations (can tolerate "partial participation"). Communications must be simple and unambiguous. Establishing trust is the most important aspect of this phase. The doctor must spend time with the patient rather than "wait for the patient to become more coherent to use therapy." This is also the best time to schedule educational meetings with family and begin providing information about medications and the course of illness.

In the stabilization phase, the following tenets of psychosocial rehabilitation are involved:

- Build social skills.
- Train techniques for stress reduction.
- Practice conflict resolution.
- Revitalize or establish a support network.
- Train families (teach knowledge about the disease, how to help).
- Teach problem-solving skills.
- Expand psychological defense styles (decrease impulsivity or avoidance).

Unlike chronic schizophrenia, cognitive processes are not generally severely disrupted in older patients with psychosis. However, cognitive enhancement therapy is the same for both older and younger patients with schizophrenia. A group curriculum to enhance cognitive function in patients with schizophrenia was developed by Hogarty and colleagues (2004), consisting of cognitive tasks such as categorization exercises, getting the gist of a message, being able to condense communications, solving real-life social dilemmas, abstracting themes from editorial pages, appraising affective and social contexts, initiating and maintaining conversations, play writing, "center stage exercises" of introducing oneself, and psychoeducational topics. This curriculum is relevant to all patients with psychosis who show profound negative symptomatology.

SUMMARY

Psychosis in the elderly usually consists of simple delusions rather than the bizarre delusions seen in schizophrenia, and shows less disorganization. Late-onset psychosis (where the first appearance is in late life) is also usually associated with affective disorder or dementia rather than with a schizophrenoform disorder. Often the presentation of psychosis is thought to be due to a primary dopamine dysfunction in the mesolimbic area of the brain, which is, in turn, strongly influenced by seratonin, acetylcholine, and other neurotransmitters. Biological activity in the brain reflects the brain's appraisal and adaptive responses to external events. For this reason, medication treatment alone is rarely sufficient to resolve psychopathology. To be effective, treatment must consider predisposing factors, redress the psychosocial precipitants, and provide psychotherapy and/or social services. The prognosis, with proper treatment, is as good as treatment for schizophrenia.

7

ANXIETY DISORDERS

Anxiety is a universal phenomenon, whereas severe or chronic anxiety is a disorder. It is also a comorbid trait with virtually all psychiatric disorders. Traditionally, anxiety is thought to be activated as a warning against potential danger, leading to either adaptive responses (fight or flight) or total disorganization when overwhelmed by stress (freezing). Anxiety is strongly linked to memory. One can often not forget traumatic incidents, and it is common to experience a flood of anxiety with every reminder of a particularly negative event.

BACKGROUND

A stress that is life threatening to self or loved ones is considered a universal catastrophic threat that would make even the hardiest person anxious, and this type of life-threatening experience is required to justify a diagnosis of a posttraumatic stress disorder (PTSD; American Psychiatric Association, 2000). All other stresses are viewed as having an element of variability due to how the individual sees it. Psychological defense mechanisms, mastery, rehearsal (exposure or inoculation), cognitive abilities and flexibility, and social supports all modify the perception of a stressful event as being a source of stress or not.

The criteria for the type of stress that can cause PTSD require two components. The first is a direct personal exposure to a catastrophic stress (actual or threatened death, serious injury, threat to one's physical integrity [e.g., rape], witnessing the death or injury of another person) or learning about death or harm to someone close. The second equally important criterion is that the person experiences intense fear, helplessness, or horror. In children, the response can be manifest by disorganized or agitated behavior (American Psychiatric Association, 2000).

The one exception to this hierarchy of stress is in cognitively impaired older adults, who might show catastrophic reactions to minimal provocation. Like children, it seems that individuals who feel helpless instinctively turn to a protector (attachment figure) and become anxious when their protector is gone (separation anxiety). Even being out of the house among strangers or in a novel setting might be perceived as a stressful event by an elderly person who is frightened to be alone.

A pioneer in the field, Hans Selye, described good and bad stress. The stress involved in pleasant events such a child's wedding is good and does not usually cause emotional disturbance or physical decline. On the other hand, negative events such as forced retirement can lead to anxiety, depression, and even cause negative health consequences (e.g., a heart attack). The original fight–flight model does not incorporate a notion of "good" or "bad" stress, or of the long-term health effects of chronic stress.

Under conditions of chronic or recurring stressors, anxiety is eventually divorced from the apparent stressor. This view is akin to the kindling model of bipolar disorder: Anxiety becomes constant, with a life of its own. It is like a fire that has been kindled and burns without further fuel from a stressful situation.

Anxiety is also intimately involved with memory acquisition and forgetting. Optimal levels of anxiety or arousal is needed for learning to occur. However, severe stress can lead to either entrenched traumatic memories, as in PTSD, or to no memory, as in dissociative states. These extreme responses are also not accommodated in the original model.

High baseline anxiety is usually thought to represent "trait anxiety." Individuals with high trait anxiety tend to overreact to stress and are unable to function under it. It is very common to hear patients say "I've always been a nervous person" when asked when problems began.

NEUROBIOLOGICAL EXPLANATION

Longstanding speculation posits that the hypothylamic–pituitary–adrenal (HPA) axis must underlie chronic stress-related effects, including immune changes, because the autonomic nervous system has a central role in mediating adaptation and immediate stress reactions.

Several interconnected pathways or circuits control anxiety. The fronto-cingulate cortex, associated with appraisal and worry, connects to subcortical areas (thalamus, amygdala, hippocampus, basal ganglia) and modulates reactions to stimuli. Pathways to the temporal lobe insular region further modulate the HPA axis and automomic reactivity. All circuits are interconnected and have feedback loops. The HPA axis is probably the most widely studied part of the associated circuits of anxiety. Better cortisol assay methods reveal new information about HPA dysregulation associated with PTSD and anxiety disorders. After trauma, diurnal variation in cortisol release seems to be lost, with constantly high-normal levels of cortisol secretion. Hippocampal neuronal cell loss is thought to result from chronic cortisol overstimulation. The risk of long-term cognitive impairment due to chronic anxiety provides additional reason for early treatment.

At the cellular level, there is relative glutamate overactivity and GABA underactivity. GABA is an inhibitory neurotransmitter, and glutamate is considered an excitatory neurotransmitter. GABA and glutamate modulate neuronal excitability and central nervous system (CNS) arousal.

There are three types of glutamate receptors: AMPA, NMDA, and G-protein-coupled receptors. The first is excitatory postsynaptic currents (EPSC), activated by AMPA-kainate-mediated fast EPSC receptors (a-amino-3-hydroxy-5-methyl-4-isoxazole propionic acid). The second is voltage-dependent NMDA receptors (N-methyl-D-aspartate). And the third is a receptor coupled to a G-protein. The fast EPSC receptors have been the main point of interest in anxiety, but the other glutamate receptors may also be involved in long-term modulation of anxiety symptoms. Corticotrophin releasing factor (CRF) and other neurotrophins modulate glutamate response. Anxiolytics currently are GABA agonists, but medications targeting glutamate and CRF function may define new treatments for pathological anxiety that may have less effect on the cholinergic system and memory.

Another potential use of biological changes is to serve as a biological marker for pathological anxiety. Although a biological marker may seem unnecessary on the surface, it is not. One often sees patients who appear severely anxious but have no awareness of it, or the converse situation of patients who appear calm but complain of incapacitating anxiety. The clinician often questions whether to treat or not and needs an external target to judge efficacy of treatment. In search of a potential blood test for anxiety disorders, an Israeli group described an index of AChE, BChE, and PON related to body mass index (BMI) that may demonstrate true anxiety disorders (Soreq, 2005).

Genes that code for the neurotransmitters and receptors involved in anxiety or panic disorder have been located on chromosomes 1, 11, and 13. These could serve as possible biological markers if pathological alleles are found that are strong predictors of anxiety disorders or can provide directions for novel treatments.

Neurotransmitters implicated in anxiety are listed in Table 7.1.

Table 7.1. Neurotransmitters Implicated in Anxiety

EXCITATORY NEUROTRANSMITTERS	INHIBITORY NEUROTRANSMITTERS	NEUROTRANSMITTERS INVOLVED IN COGNITION
L-glutamic acid	GABA$_A$ related to anxiety*	Acetylcholine
L-homocysteic acid	GABA$_B$ related to	Dopamine (D$_1$ receeptors
L-aspartic acid	depression*	in the frontal brain
L-cysteine sulfate		regions)
L-serine-O-sulfate		
Quinolinic acid		
Norepinephrine		
Dopamine		

GABA is enhanced by anticonvulsants and tricyclic antidepressants.

NORMAL VERSUS ABNORMAL BEHAVIOR

There are limited data in the literature about different anxiety disorders in older adults. Most publications are general review articles or SSRI efficacy studies. Overall clinical impressions about anxiety disorders in older adults are listed in Table 7.2.

Table 7.2. DSM-IV Anxiety Disorders in Older Adults

Panic Attack Panic Disorder without agoraphobia (300.01) Panic Disorder with agoraphobia (300.21)	Only one in four elderly with panic disorder will admit it. Panic is often inferred by refusal to be left alone and suggestive medical symptoms. Often the person wants only one particular individual to be near, such as a spouse (attachment figure). Agoraphobia is relatively rare in elderly.
Agoraphobia without History of Panic (300.22)	Agoraphobia is relatively rare in elderly but fear of falling is common (rule out vestibular abnormalities).
Social Phobia (300.23)	Generally a young person's disorder. When it occurs in elderly, it is often related to embarrassment due to inability to recall names or being ashamed of appearance due to illness.
Specific Phobia (300.29)	Most common phobias appear to be • Fear of death • Fear of disaster to family • Dental anxiety
Obsessive–Compulsive Disorder (300.3)	The most common forms in elderly are • Compulsive hoarding • Obsessions about health (including compulsive handwashing) • Remorse about an old transgression (such as a spouse learning about a marital infidelity 30 years earlier) • Rare—need for symmetry or counting.
Posttraumatic Stress Disorder (309.81)	Cardinal symptoms are reexperiencing, avoidance, and hyperarousal. Elderly often have more hyperarousal symptoms than younger adults. Trauma reactivation 30 years or more after an event has been described, speculatively due to helplessness related to onset of disability or specific cues that revive old memories.

Table 7.2. (continued)

Acute Stress Disorder (308.30)	No references to elderly were found on Medline.
Generalized Anxiety Disorder (GAD; 300.02)	Almost 50% of GAD progresses to depression within 3 years.
Anxiety Disorder Due to [indicate the General Medical Condition] (293.84)	Reports most often around vestibular dysfunction or medication induced
Substance-Induced Anxiety Disorder (292.89, specify substance)	No references to elderly were found on Medline.
Anxiety Disorder Not Otherwise Specified (300.00)	No references to elderly were found on Medline.

UNIQUE ASPECTS OF THE DISORDER IN ELDERLY

The landmark NIMH Epidemiologic Catchment Area (ECA) study completed 25 years ago showed an unexpectedly low prevalence of anxiety disorders in older adults. This finding did not match the general observation that anxiety complaints in the elderly population seem higher than in younger patients. This discrepancy is explained by the fact that anxiety in older adults commonly coexists with other psychiatric or medical disorders and is not listed as an independent diagnosis. Agoraphobia (fear of being in a place or situation from which escape might be difficult, leading to avoidance of public events or travel) may not occur as frequently in the elderly, and episodes of anxiety may not reach the criteria of a full-blown panic attack.

ASSESSMENT AND DIAGNOSIS

It is important to ascertain (1) the level of trait anxiety (general reaction to stress), (2) the initial precipitant to see if it was a catastrophic event or a negative appraisal of a more minor event, (3) if panic attacks occur, and (4) the frequency of symptoms. Because anxiety symptoms often coexist with depression or other psychiatric disorders, other diagnoses should be considered if anxiety exists.

Aside from extreme stressors that could lead to PTSD, the most common "geriatric stressors" that often lead to anxiety in older adults seem to be:

- Loss (death of a loved one, worries about children or spouse)
- Fear of dependency
  - ✓ Fear of losing one's house and being relocated
  - ✓ Fear of being unable to afford rent or medicines
  - ✓ Fear of chronic illness and disability (even from hypertension)
  - ✓ Fear of falling
- Fear of victimization (even by children taking assets)
- Family conflicts
- Retirement
- Fear of death
- Role reversal

TREATMENT METHODS

Medications

SSRIs and SNRIs have become preferred agents for almost all anxiety disorders. In general, benzodiazepines are avoided in the elderly population, especially in frail older adults or those with cognitive impairment, due to the risk of falls and increased confusion. However, if benzodiazepines are needed, it seems best to use an intermediate-acting one without active metabolites, such as lorazepam or alprazolam, at low doses. Long-acting benzodiazepines with active metabolites, such as clonazepam, diazepam, or chlordiazepoxide, should be avoided. In making a change from a medication such as clonazepam to other medications, taper off over 1–2 weeks to avoid rebound anxiety.

Based on studies with younger adults, medication management of anxiety disorders has shifted from benzodiazepine monotherapy ($GABA_A$ receptor agonism) to antidepressant monotherapy, mainly SSRIs or SNRIs. Anticonvulsants have been used selectively, especially gabapentin or tiagabine, due to actions on the GABA system. Research on new medications involve glutamate inhibitors, alpha-2-delta ligands, and CRF1 antagonists that are not commercially available. The duration of treatment is not standardized but usually extends to at least 6 months after remission of symptoms, provided there has been adequate removal of stressors and improvement in coping abilities.

The only exception to when benzodiazepines are acceptable as first choice is when short-term use is anticipated (e.g., as a rescue medication when starting an SSRI or during an acute period of stress). Patients should be alerted to the fact that benzodiazepines should be temporary and should not be needed once the main problem, such as a depression, improves. An intermediate-acting benzodiazepine such as lorazepam would be preferred over longer-acting medications with active metabolites to reduce adverse effects. Doses should be minimized.

Limited data exist for use of mood stabilizers, although case reports show benefit. However, because of limited data, these remain tertiary choices at this time. Atypical antipsychotics are increasingly used as an adjunct, but not as a primary treatment, for any anxiety disorder. However, limited data for using atypical antipsychotics for anxiety in the elderly dictate that this approach should also remain a tertiary treatment choice.

Psychosocial Interventions

Because of the heterogeneous list of causes for anxiety disorders, it is best to say that one matches the psychotherapy with the person. No double-blind or comparative treatment study has been attempted regarding different psychotherapy models for treating anxiety in older adults. Although treatment approaches appear eclectic, they generally follow this sequence:

- Teach palliative or distractive techniques (e.g., relaxation exercises, meditation, soothing thoughts).
- Use cognitive–behavioral therapy (CBT) next to help the patient gain control over specific symptoms. Problem-solving skills, guided imagery, and active rather than passive coping styles are emphasized. Psychotherapies aimed at teaching relaxation skills, improving understanding of the precipitating circumstances (psychoeducation), improving coping

skills, and restoring or building a support network are critical for most patients.

- Use expressive therapies (psychodynamic psychotherapies) to gain understanding of reasons for treatment resistance, to encourage abreaction and release of suppressed emotion/ anger in some cases, or to resolve longstanding conflictual issues that underlie the present problems.

Group therapy approaches often appear especially helpful in anxiety disorders, even for older adults who say they eschew groups. An algorithm for treatment options is summarized in Table 7.3 from the literature and from personal experience.

Table 7.3. Treatment Options for Anxiety Disorders in Older Adults

DSM-IV DIAGNOSIS	MEDICATION CATEGORY	PSYCHOTHERAPY APPROACHES (can be individual or group)
Panic Attack Panic Disorder without Agoraphobia (300.01) Panic Disorder with Agoraphobia (300.21)	First—SSRI Second—TCA Third—benzodiazepines Fourth—MAOIs Fifth—other antide-pressants (from APA Panic Disorder Practice Guideline)	First —palliative and distraction techniques —relaxation training, meditation —information and social services —supportive therapy Second—CBT Third—expressive therapies
Agoraphobia without History of Panic (300.22)	Assume treatment similar to other phobias	Assume treatment similar to other phobias
Social Phobia (300.23) Not common in elderly	SNRI (venlafaxine*) or SSRI (sertraline, paroxetine*)	Behavioral therapy (exposure and response prevention) or CBT are usually described
Specific Phobia (300.29)	SNRI (venlafaxine*) or SSRI (sertraline, paroxetine*)	Behavioral therapy (exposure and response prevention) or CBT are usually described

Table 7.3. (continued)

DSM-IV DIAGNOSIS	MEDICATION CATEGORY	PSYCHOTHERAPY APPROACHES (can be individual or group)
Obsessive–Compulsive Disorder (300.3)	First—SSRI (fluoxetine, sertraline, paroxetine, celexa, fluvoxamine*) Second—TCA Third—SNRI	Behavioral therapy (exposure and response prevention) or CBT are usually described
Posttraumatic Stress Disorder (309.81)	Immediately after trauma: —benzodiazepines (short term, prn) —hypnotics for sleep (short term, prn) After diagnosis: First—SSRI (sertraline and paroxetine*) Second—TCA (imipramine studied) Third—MAOI (phenelzine studied) Adjunct: A novel antipsychotic (olanzapine studied) Benzodiazepines have not been effective. Other antidepressant classes have not been studied systematically.	After trauma (first 3 months): First—education, information, supportive measures Second—palliative and distraction techniques, such as relaxation training and meditation, and information and social services. After diagnosis (about 6 months): First—education and supportive measures Second—CBT Third—No specific research
Acute Stress Disorder (308.30)	Assume same as PTSD	Assume same as PTSD
Generalized Anxiety Disorder (300.02)	First—SSRI or buspirone Second—SNRI Third—gabapentin, tiagabine, pregabalin	First —palliative and distraction techniques —relaxation training, meditation —information and social services —supportive therapy Second—CBT Third—expressive therapies

Table 7.3. (continued)

DSM-IV DIAGNOSIS	MEDICATION CATEGORY	PSYCHOTHERAPY APPROACHES (can be individual or group)
Anxiety Disorder Not Otherwise Specified (300.00)	No specific recommendation; probably best to follow GAD algorithm	First —palliative and distraction techniques —relaxation training, meditation —information and social services —supportive therapy Second—CBT Third—expressive therapies
Substance-Induced Anxiety Disorder (292.89, specify substance)	Probably best to use a novel antipsychotic at low doses (with some exception, benzodiazepines may be preferable)	First —palliative and distraction techniques —relaxation training, meditation —information and social services Second—support groups

* These have FDA indications for this diagnosis. SSRI = serotonin specific reuptake inhibitor; TCA = tricyclic antidepressant; MAOI = monoamine oxidase inhibitor; SNRI = (selective) serotonin norepinephrine reuptake inhibitor; GAD = generalized anxiety disorder; CBT = cognitive–behavioral therapy; PTSD = posttraumatic stress disorder.

Optimal treatment of anxiety disorders in older adults requires application of the biopsychosocial model. Medications are used to reduce the most severe symptoms and improve sleep (biological); environmental interventions are used to decrease chronic threats (remove perpetuating factors) and provide psychotherapy aimed at improving problem-solving and coping techniques, rebuilding the social support network, and increasing understanding of the disorder (i.e., build buffers and lessen the appraisal of risk).

CASE EXAMPLE

Mrs. A is an 84-year-old widow living in a life-care community in New Orleans after Hurricane Katrina. She endured an evac-

uation and 3-month hiatus to a crowded nursing home in Baton
Rouge. Staff turnover rates in both facilities was very high. She
was referred for psychiatric evaluation because she became acutely
forgetful, complained of difficulty falling asleep, was frequently
awoken by nightmares, and extremely irritable. She denied excessive worry, but appeared anxious and fidgety with poor attention.

Before the hurricane, the patient showed mild cognitive
impairment. While her appraisal of the situation in New
Orleans after Katrina was not one of intense fear or horror, she
experienced the type of stress sufficient to cause PTSD (learning about the "threatened death" of people who refused to leave,
and being inundated with news of the destruction of her city).
Upon returning to New Orleans the patient felt everything was
different; her family was no longer close enough to visit. She
had been on diazepam (Valium) for over 30 years, prescribed
by her doctor, though she denied any psychiatric problems.

Treatment involved switching from a benzodiazepine,
which might worsen her memory complaint, to an SSRI. This
took considerable psychoeducation and coaxing for patient
compliance. Use of short-term palliative measures was provided (relaxation training, asking her about her family,
requesting social services, and giving her a timetable for when
she could expect a full restoration of services). Further exposure
and response prevention in a CBT treatment was not needed.

The patient reported less irritability, seemed less forgetful,
and showed less manifest anxiety or sleep complaints within a
month. PTSD never appeared. Even at age 84, the patient's
appraisal of the situation was not one of intense fear or helplessness, even though she may have had a predisposition for it with
a history of "anxious personality" that required sedatives for
much of her adult life. An SSRI was given, despite the mildness
of her symptoms, to treat the biological origins of her symptoms
and in order to eliminate benzodiazepines. The most important
intervention was instilling hope and a sense of security.

SUMMARY

Anxiety is a signal or warning for a potentially dangerous situation
in older populations. Premorbid dispositions, such as genetics and

learned experiences, can turn normal reactions to stress into a disease process. Per the DSM-IV, there is a spectrum of anxiety disorders and anxiety-related manifestations, and a combination of psychosocial and medication approaches is usually effective. Non-medication, supportive approaches are ideal for older patients.

8

SLEEP DISORDERS

The International Classification of Sleep Disorders divides insomnia into the following three major categories (American Academy of Sleep Medicine, 2001):

- Dyssomnias
  - ✓ Intrinsic sleep disturbance (primary insomnia)
  - ✓ Extrinsic sleep disturbance (e.g., due to habits such as naps)
  - ✓ Circadian rhythm sleep disorders (e.g., sleep advance)
- Parasomnias
  - ✓ Arousal disorders (e.g., sleepwalking)
  - ✓ Sleep–wake transition disorders (e.g., nocturnal leg cramps)
  - ✓ Parasomnias associated with REM sleep (e.g., nightmares)
  - ✓ Other parasomnias (e.g., bruxism)
- Sleep disorders associated with mental, neurological, and other medical disorders (e.g., sleep apnea)

This chapter focuses primarily on dyssomnias (disturbance in the normal rhythm or pattern of sleep) such as insomnia and sleep-phase disturbance. Parasomnias (disorders that interfere with sleep) such as sleep apnea, restless leg syndrome, and bruxism (teeth grinding when asleep) and other medical problems causing sleep disturbance are important to recognize because they occur most commonly in the elderly population. These are mainly medical problems that require medical interventions rather than hypnotics, treatment of a primary psychiatric disorder, or behavioral interventions.

Often sleep complaints reflect normal changes in sleep architecture or poor sleep hygiene, such as naps. Patients often insist on medications for sleep and doctors are usually happy to comply, although the elderly are more prone to adverse effects from sleeping medications than younger age groups.

BACKGROUND

Almost half of all adults in the United States complain of insomnia (Gallup, 1995.) In fact, sleep complaints are possibly the most common complaint that a general physician encounters in practice. Elderly patients routinely complain about interrupted sleep (frequent awakenings) and sleep advance problems (going to bed too early and getting up too early). This pattern may not be abnormal, because deep stages of sleep decrease and frequent awakenings occur even in normal older adults. Differentiating pathological from normal sleep patterns in this population is especially important because they may be (1) due to neurological problems such as sleep apnea, (2) a sign of depression or delirium, or (3) a side effect of a medication.

NEUROBIOLOGICAL EXPLANATION

Sleep appears to be regulated by a wake-promoting area in the posterior hypothalamus and a sleep-promoting region in the preoptic area (circadian "clock"). The balance between these two areas produces sleep cycles wherein each has its own diurnal rhythm and peak effects at different times. When the wake-promoting area predominates, we feel alert; when the sleep-promoting area predominates, we cannot stay awake. However, body rhythms are influenced by stress and other environmental cues (Saper et al., 2001).

$GABA_A$ benzodiazepine agonists have been the main targets for hypnotics, but other neurotransmitters or peptides, including serotonin, norepinephrine, melatonin, histamine, and acetylcholine, are involved in sleep regulation.

Light seems to be a major influence in setting circadian rhythms mediated by melatonin. This hormone (5-methoxy-N-acetyltryptamine) is produced by the pineal gland and retina, and is influenced by bright light exposure akin to daylight (2,000 lux). Melatonin is synthesized from the amino acid L-tryptophan (a precursor of serotonin). In older adults melatonin secretion seems to be of shorter duration and peaks at different times. Sleep-phase advance seems correlated with a peaking of melatonin earlier in the day.

In central sleep apnea, the central medullary-pontine respiratory drive is abnormal. The trigger to breathe in a rhythmic fashion and maintain O_2 homeostasis is no longer functional, and the trigger to breath resorts to CO_2 buildup (hypercapnea). This brainstem dysfunction is associated with severe illness such as stroke, congestive heart failure, CNS infection, bulbar degeneration, and high cervical spinal surgery complications (National Institute of Neurological Disorders and Stroke, 2007). The more common form of sleep apnea is due to external obstruction of the airway, and requires measures to free airflow.

The basis of restless leg syndrome (RLS) is unknown. There is a family history of RLS in 50% of patients, but a genetic link has not been demonstrated. The substantia nigra and striatum that mediate smooth, purposeful movements are the likely areas to be impaired, based on symptoms, and dopmamine the main neurotransmitter (National Institute of Neurological Disorders and Stroke, 2007).

NORMAL VERSUS ABNORMAL BEHAVIOR

Normal sleep patterns in the elderly involve lighter sleep (less of Stages 3 and 4), but contrary to common opinion, not more or less sleep. Awakenings during the night become common but are still considered normal if the patient can fall back to sleep without much effort. Often there is a mild sleep-phase advance (getting sleepy earlier). In general, it is common for older adults to awaken two or three times per night but fall asleep quickly and feel rested during the day. Rapid eye movement (REM) patterns do not seem to change with age, though the cycles occur a little less frequently.

In EEG studies, sleep has been divided into five stages, one REM and four non-REM (nREM) stages (Kwentus, 2004):

- nREM Stage 1—drowsiness (EEG background rhythm is about 6 Hz)
- nREM Stage 2—light sleep
- NREM Stages 3 and 4—deep sleep (EEG background rhythm is about 2–4 Hz, with K complexes high-amplitude triphasic waves, and sleep spindles; bursts of 12–14 Hz activity)
- REM Stage 5—typically lasts 10 minutes (EEG speeds up, muscle tone is low causing virtual paralysis)

In younger adults, sleep goes in 60- to 90-minute cycles starting at Stage 1, progressing to Stage 4, going backward to Stage 2, and then to REM. The cycles are usually repeated without awakening. In older adults, deep stages of sleep are often shorter or lost, the percentage of REM decreases, and Stage 2 predominates (Leventhal & Burns, 2004).

As noted, sleep-phase advance is often seen in older adults. They go to bed right after dinner (6 or 7 P.M.) and awaken 8 hours later (2 to 3 A.M.), fully rested.

Insomnia occurs in 30–50% of chronic medical diseases such as diabetes, myocardial infarctions, congestive heart failure, angina, hip pain, prostate disease, and obstructive pulmonary disease (Katz, 1998). It is also occurs in up to 40% of psychiatric disorders, especially anxiety, major depression (Ford & Kamerow, 1989), and delirium. Because of the high frequency of insomnia in these disorders, it can often be used as an early marker of relapse.

Sleep apnea is classically divided into obstructive and central sleep apnea. The symptomatic hallmark of obstructive sleep apnea is usually obesity, snoring, and chronic daytime fatigue. Chronic sleep deprivation also leads to irritability and memory complaints. Diagnosis is made on polysomnography. The pause in breathing must last 10 seconds to be considered apnea (six breaths/minute). Central sleep apnea is differentiated from obstructive sleep apnea by whether breathing stops (central) or movements of breathing continue (chest movement), but airflow at the nose and mouth stop. Moderately severe apnea shows a pause of 15–30 seconds, and severe, greater than 30 seconds between some breaths.

Bruxism is related to tension and aggressive, overcompetetive tendencies. It is diagnosed by excessive wearing of the tips of the teeth on dental examination.

RLS may account for 10% of chronic insomnia. The syndrome has also been called periodic limb movement disorder (PLMD), the Ekbom syndrome, the Wittmaack–Ekbom syndrome, and anxietas tibialis. It is diagnosed by a desire to move the limbs, often accompanied by paresthesia (numbness) or dysesthesia (altered sensation). Symptoms occur only at rest where motor restlessness and nocturnal worsening occur and are alleviated by activity. As noted, 50% of cases have a family history of RLS, which is associated with diverse medical disorders and is relieved when the causal disorder is corrected. For example, RLS is associated with low iron levels or anemia, uremia, Parkinson's disease, peripheral neuropathy, diabetes, late pregnancies (last trimester), malignancy, smoking, excessive caffeine intake, antipsychotics, antileptics, and antinausea medications. When any of those causes is corrected, RLS improves. Caffeine, alcohol and tobacco may aggravate or trigger symptoms in those predisposed to RLS. Although associated with parkinsonism and helped by an anti-Parkinson's medication, the disorder does not appear to progress to Parkinson's disease (i.e., it is not a prodromal symptom; National Institute of Neurological Disorders and Stroke, 2007).

UNIQUE ASPECTS OF THE DISORDER IN ELDERLY

Medical illness usually leads to discomfort or inability to stay asleep (interrupted sleep). Medication-induced insomnia, such as the use of activating medications, or substance withdrawal (such as from alcohol, benzodiazepine, or pain medication) are other common causes of insomnia. Intrinsic sleep disturbances, such as sleep apnea, and sleep–wake transition disorders, such as RLS, seem more common in late life. The causes must be considered first because medical management or treatment of the primary cause, such as antidepressants for depressive insomnia, is the definitive treatment.

ASSESSMENT AND DIAGNOSIS

The phase in which sleep problems occur (early, middle, or late) is one of the more important clues to the diagnosis. Insomnia related to anxiety and stress usually causes problems falling asleep. Sleep disturbance related to depression usually leads to middle and late insomnia (frequent awakenings and early morning rising). Medical disorders usually affect the capacity to stay asleep due to discomfort. Often spouses must give information about whether the patient snores or seems to stop breathing for long periods. Table 8.1 lists the common patterns that cause sleep problems.

Table 8.1. Common Patterns of Sleep Problems

SLEEP PHASE	FREQUENCY	DURATION	POTENTIAL CAUSE
Early (sleep onset)	Transient	Short term (< 3 weeks)	Situational stress (e.g., bereavement, relocation, finances) Sleep hygiene (sleep schedule change, noise, light, stimulant use) Sleep-phase disturbance
Middle (interrupted sleep)	Persistent (nightly)	Months to years	Protracted stress Medical cause • Physical discomfort (e.g., pain or nocturia) • Sleep apnea • Restless leg syndrome
Mixed (early and middle insomnia)	Persistent (nightly)	Months to years	Protracted stress Medical cause • Physical discomfort • Other sleep disorder
Late (early morning rising)	Persistent (nightly)	Months to years	Depression

The patterns of insomnia in older adults suggest a stronger likelihood of stress-related insomnia, poor sleep hygiene, medical causes, and depression, rather than primary insomnia, and often require treatments other than sedative hypnotics. Useful questions to determine sleep hygiene are listed in Table 8.2.

Table 8.2. Questions to Ask about Sleep Hygiene

What is your typical bedtime? Is it the same time every night?
Are you sleepy when you go to bed?
Do you use your bedroom for anything but sleep?
Do you nap or rest during the day? When? Where? How long?
Do you have a relaxation period before retiring?
Do you experience tension in your muscles or anxiety when you fall asleep?
Do you exercise within 4 hours of going to bed?
What medications do you use?
Do you use caffeinated drinks, smoke, or drink alcohol before going to sleep?
Do you use an alarm to awaken at the same time every morning?
Keep a sleep diary for 2 weeks and record:
  • Total sleep time (subjective)
  • Actual time entering and leaving bed
  • Time to fall asleep (subjective)
  • Number of awakenings during the night
  • Time to fall asleep again after waking
  • Time of final awakening (even if you stay in bed trying to sleep later)
If there is an informant, ask about
  • Snoring
  • Appears to stop breathing?
  • Confirmation of sleep quality (e.g., frequent awakenings, gets out of bed, appears to have nightmares)

Sleep labs should be used when suspicion of a parasomnia, requiring medical intervention, exists.

TREATMENT METHODS

Before considering medications, removal of potential causes for insomnia must be attempted. Sleep disturbances secondary to psychiatric illness or medical illness need to be addressed by primary attention to treatment of the medical or psychiatric disorder, with the possible need for short-term hypnotics, as already discussed. Pain management is often an important intervention. Patients with pain often say their sleeping pill is acetaminophen (Tylenol). Geriatric patients should be discouraged from taking Tylenol-PM, however, because it contains diphenhydramine, which may cause confusion or falls.

If a person is on an off-label medication for sleep that can cause more confusion or unsteadiness, such as diphenhydramine or clonazepam, or is on trazadone or quetiapine for a primary insomnia, slow tapering or every-other-day dosing (to allow slow discontinuation of the medication without significant rebound insomnia) is recommended. Appropriate sleep interventions can then be addressed.

For sleep-phase advance, bright light exposure in the late afternoon may delay peak production of melatonin and help the patient fall asleep later and awaken at a more reasonable morning hour.

Medications and Medical Interventions

Medications used for insomnia fall into three main categories:

- Benzodiazepines
  - ✓ Class that is typically approved for treatment of insomnia (note that lorazepam or clonazepam are not approved)
- Nonbenzodiazepine hypnotics—for example, zolpidem, escopiclone, rameleton
- Alternatives used in common practice (off-label use)
  - ✓ Antihistamines (over-the-counter)
  - ✓ Herbal therapies
  - ✓ Antidepressants (without depression)—for example, trazadone, amitriptyline
  - ✓ Antipsychotics (without psychosis)—for example, quetiapine

Because of an increased risk of cognitive impairment, falls, and daytime somnolence due to slower metabolism, medications for insomnia with older patients should have an FDA indication for sleep, and should be selected on the basis of avoidance of adverse effects, assuming equal efficacy. There are no comparative trials of hypnotics for older adults, so the principles of geriatric medication selection and prescribing should be applied.

Figure 8.1 shows why it is important to know the t_{max} and $t_{1/2}$ (half-life) of hypnotics, which also appear on Tables 8.3 and 8.4. Speed of onset of is predicted by t_{max} and duration of effect is predicted by the half-life and whether there are active metabolites. Patients should not be subjected to a medication hangover in the morning, which they would experience with long-acting medications. Except for ramelteon, which binds to melatonin receptors, nonbenzodiazepine agents are scheduled medications that act on the $GABA_A$ receptor complex, although distant from the benzodiazepine and barbiturate receptor sites. They have the advantage of having less A.M. drowsiness and less abuse potential than tranquilizers. Time-release forms of short-acting hypnotics allow fewer awakenings but theoretically increase the risk of morning sedation due to the delayed release of medication.

Tables 8.3 and 8.4 provide overviews of the pharmacokinetic properties of benzodiazepine and nonbenzodiazepine medications used for sleep disturbances.

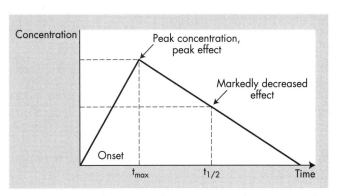

Figure 8.1. Linear absorption and excretion curves (not exponential). Slopes differ for each medication.

Table 8.3. Pharmacokinetic Properties of Benzodiazepines
Used for Sleep Disturbances

MEDICATION	DOSE (range)	ONSET (hr.)	HALF-LIFE (hr.)
Estazolam (ProSomm)	2 mg (0.5–2 mg)	Slow (T_{max} 2)	12–15
Flurazepam (Dalmane)	15 mg (7.5–30 mg)	Rapid (T_{max} 1)	6–8
Quazepam (Doral)	15 mg (7.5–30 mg)	Intermediate (T_{max} 1.5)	39–73
Temazepam (Restoril)	15 mg (7.5–30 mg)	Intermediate (T_{max} 1.5)	10–15
Triazolam (Halcion)	0.25 mg (0.125–0.5 mg)	Rapid (T_{max} 1)	1.5–5.5
OFF-LABEL			
Lorazepam (Ativan)	1 mg (0.5–2 mg)	Intermediate (T_{max} 1.5)	12
Diazepam (Valium)	2 mg (2–10 mg)	Slow (T_{max} 2)	20–50; metabolite 30–200
Chlordiazepoxide (Librium)	5 mg (5–25 mg)	Slow (T_{max} 0.5–4)	24–48; metabolite 21–78
Clonazepam (Klonopin)	1 mg 0.4–1.5 mg (< 20 mg)	Slow (T_{max} 1–4)	30–40

*Note. PDR dose ranges. Kinetics are approximate; ranges vary widely (1 hour or more).
BZ = benzodiazepine.*

Table 8.3. (continued)

AWAKENINGS	RECEPTOR	ACTIVE METABOLITES	RENAL ADJUSTMENT	CYP PATHWAY
Reduced	Ω1 receptor agonist	Yes	Not studied	3A4
Reduced	Type 3 BZ	Yes	No	3A4
Reduced	Type 1 BZ receptor	Yes	Not studied	Not specified
Reduced	Ω1 receptor agonist (sleep), W2 (anxiety) BZ receptors	No	No	Conjugation, no significant oxidative path
Unchanged	Type 1 BZ	No	No	3A4
OFF-LABEL				
Reduced	BZ receptors	No	No	Glucuronidation, no significant oxidative path
Reduced	BZ receptors	Yes	Yes	3A4, 2C19
Reduced	BZ receptors	Yes	Yes	3A4
Reduced	BZ receptors	No	No	3A4

Table 8.4. Pharmacokinetic Properties of Nonbenzodiazepines
Used for Sleep Disturbances

MEDICATION	DOSE (Range)	ONSET (hr.)	HALF-LIFE (hr.)
Zolpidem (Ambien)	5 mg (5–10 mg)	Rapid (T_{max} 1.5)	2.5
Zolpidem (Ambien CR)	6.25 mg (6.25–12.5 mg)	Biphasic (T_{max} 1.5)	2.8
Zaleplon (Sonata)	5 mg (5–20 mg)	Rapid (T_{max} 1)	1
Eszopicione (Lunesta)	1 mg (1–3 mg)	Rapid (T_{max} 1)	6
Rameleton (Rozerem)	8 mg	Rapid (T_{max} 0.75)	1–2.6

Table 8.4. (continued)

AWAKENINGS	RECEPTOR	ACTIVE METABOLITES	RENAL ADJUSTMENT	HEPATIC ADJUSTMENT
Reduced	$GABA_A$	No	No	Reduce dose 50%
Reduced	$GABA_A$	No	No	Reduce dose 50%
Reduced	$GABA_A$ Low $\Omega 1$ and $\Omega 2$	No	No	Reduce dose (70% less clearance); 3A4; aldehyde oxidase
Reduced	$GABA_A$	No	No	Reduce dose (50% less clearance), 3A4, 2E1
Unchanged	Melatonin MT1, MT2	No	No	Don't use 1A2, 2C9, 3A4

Off-label use of psychotropics or antihistamines for primary insomnia is not indicated for the reasons listed in Table 8.5.

Table 8.5. Problems with Off-Label Psychotropics or Antihistamines for Primary Insomnia

AGENT	PROBLEM
Trazadone (Desyrel)	Uncertain dosing
	No studies demonstrating efficacy
	Priapism (mainly in younger men)
	Daytime sedation
Quetiapine (Seroquel) or other antipsychotics	Uncertain dosing
	No demonstrated efficacy
	Side effects
	Cost
Clonazepam (Klonopin)	Cognitive side effects
	Daytime sedation
Diphenhydramine (Benadryl)	Confusion
	Falls
Tricyclics (e.g., amitriptyline)	No defined hypnotic dose
	Limited studies for primary insomnia
	Side effects
SSRI (e.g., Paxil)	No defined hypnotic dose
	Limited studies for primary insomnia
	Side effects

Obstructive sleep apnea requires the involvement of sleep specialists for sleep lab confirmation and supervision of nasal continuous positive airway pressure (CPAP) or more invasive interventions. Partial airway obstruction causing awakening is treated by weight loss, sleeping on one's side, and using CPAP or other appliances designed to keep the airway open (e.g., a mandibular repositioning device or tongue retaining device are sometimes helpful). CPAP is a mask-like device and pump that is worn every night to increase the air pressure when breathing and to keep the airway open. In extreme cases surgery may be needed, such as a uvulopalatopharyngoplasty or treacheostomy (Reite et al., 2002)

Treatment for central sleep apnea is often related to medical illness, such as congestive heart failure. If a sedative hypnotic is desired, use the shortest-acting one (currently zolpidem) and monitor O_2 saturation with a pulse oximeter after the first dose to be sure the medication does not cause worsening of hypoxia (Reite et al., 2002).

Sleep-phase advance may be reversed by exogenous melatonin, light exposure therapy in the A.M. (2,000 lux intensity, exposure for 60 minutes), as well as entrainment by fixed sleep schedules.

In most cases, bruxism can be treated effectively by training patients how to relieve discomfort on the jaw by positioning, using a specially fitting mouthpiece, or using biofeedback to relieve muscle tension in the jaw and mouth.

For RLS, dopaminergic agents used in Parkinson's disease have traditionally been the primary treatment, but the only medication approved for treatment of RLS by the FDA thus far is ropinorol (Requip). This should be started at a dose of 0.25 mg qhs for relatively severe symptoms (about 15 awakenings/week; about 2/night; U.S. Food and Drug Administration, 2006).

Psychosocial Interventions

Poor sleep hygiene is probably the major cause of primary insomnia in older adults. Habits such as going to bed when not tired, associating the bedroom with waking activities, taking daytime naps, and taking stimulants close to bedtime (e.g., caffeine, nicotine) do not foster efficient sleep.

With primary insomnia, it is important to try to reverse poor sleep hygiene before using sedative hypnotics. Use of cognitive–behavioral therapy (CBT) to alter sleep habits has been reported to be as useful as hypnotics for improving primary insomnia (Jacobs et al., 2004). Techniques that should be taught include:

- Use the bedroom primarily for sleep (associate the bedroom with sleeping).
- Prepare the bedroom for sleep (dark, quiet).
- Learn muscle relaxation, breathing, and mental focusing techniques to use during the day and at bedtime.
- Go to bed only when drowsy.
- If unable to sleep within 20–30 minutes, get out of bed and go to another room to do something relaxing (e.g., listen to music, read).
- Take no daytime naps (keep a sleep diary).

- Take no stimulants after dinner (often need to review with the patient).

As with any behavioral intervention, it is extremely difficult to alter counterproductive bedtime rituals or daytime napping. This difficulty is usually why a structured CBT model is needed.

SUMMARY

Almost half the adult population in the United States complains of insomnia. In the elderly, reduced deep sleep stages (frequent awakenings but falling back to sleep quickly) and sleep phase advance (going to bed too early and getting up early) are often mistaken for primary insomnia. Insomnia caused by depression is typically characterized by going to bed late and experiencing excessive daytime fatigue. The treatment of insomnia depends on the etiology. Hypnotics, sleep hygiene, and CBT (cognitive–behavioral therapy) are all possible treatments for primary insomnia and sleep phase changes; weight loss and continuous positive airway pressure (CPAP) for obstructive sleep apnea; antidepressants for affective sleep disturbance; and medical care for insomnia caused by chronic illness. In all instances, avoid off-label medications or long-acting benzodiazepines for treating insomnia.

Following is a summary of treatment steps or general rules to follow when addressing sleep disturbances in older adults:

- Use short- to intermediate-acting hypnotics.
- Avoid hypnotics with active metabolites.
- Be cautious with hepatic or renal impairment.
- Use nonbenzodiazepine hypnotics to reduce risk of dependence.
- Avoid off-label medications for insomnia unless all indicated medications have failed (generally refer to a sleep specialist first).
- Treat primary etiology (e.g., depression, medical diagnosis) to avoid long-term use of hypnotics.
- Treat sleep hygiene problems through CBT to avoid long-term use of hypnotics.
- Refer to a sleep lab when unable to help.

9

SOMATOFORM DISORDERS

"The common feature of somatoform disorders is the presence of physical symptoms that suggest a general medical condition (hence, the term *somatoform*) and are not fully explained by a general medical condition, by the direct effects of a substance, or by another mental disorder (e.g., mood disorder, anxiety disorder, sleep disorder, or psychotic disorder)" (American Psychiatric Association, 2000). It does not include factitious disorder (300.19), which involves a conscious fabrication of symptoms. In general medical practices, a quarter to half of the presentations are not well explained by general medical conditions (Mayou et al., 2005).

Guidelines from the DSM-IV-TR (Appendix A, American Psychiatric Association, 2000) suggest the following steps:

- Look for an associated general medical condition first, with or without psychological factors that might affect the medical condition.
- Consider the possibility of a factitious disorder if there are external incentives (secondary gain).
- Consider one of the major somatoform disorders.

The classic somatoform disorders, such as somatization disorder (300.81), conversion disorder (300.11), hypochondriasis (300.7), and body dysmorphic disorder (300.7), are only a small part of the "mind–body" duality that psychiatrists are expected to treat. It is no longer controversial to say that social stresses and psychiatric factors influence disease processes, and that physical diseases can cause psychiatric symptoms. Figure 9.1 shows the conceptual overlap between social, medical, and psychiatric disabilities.

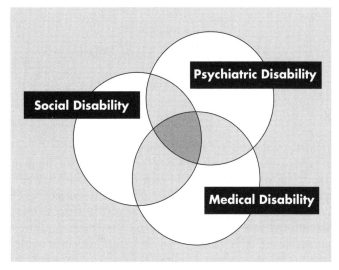

Figure 9.1. The overlapping shaded area represents somatoform disorders with varying influences from social, psychiatric, and medical issues.

This chapter is divided into two sections to highlight the differences between classic somatoform disorders and a general medical condition with or without underlying psychological factors, such as asthma, gastrointestinal distress, pain syndromes, fibromyalgia, chronic fatigue syndrome, and other stress related illnesses. Psychiatric problems as a reaction to illness, such as adjustment disorders or "reactive depressions", have been addressed in other chapters. The following case illustrates a general medical condition (adverse effects of medication) with psychological factors that might affect the medical problems.

CASE EXAMPLE

Ms. A is a 65-year-old woman with a longstanding history of schizophrenia. Although she denies hallucinations, she shows persecutory delusions, significant thought blocking, judgment problems, mutism, disorientation, and concentration difficulty. She gained excessive weight after being changed to a novel antipsychotic when early signs of tardive dyskinesia were noted from years of phenothiazine and haloperidol exposure. She is markedly obese with noninsulin-dependent diabetes, hypertension, COPD from years of smoking, and cardiomegally with mild congestive heart failure. She has become preoccupied with fears of a fatal disease, and her limited communication is restricted to multiple vague physical complaints. She has become noncompliant with treatment because she believes that one of her medications is a poison, and she cannot follow dietary restrictions. Siblings are only peripherally involved, and the patient has no husband or children. Primary complaints are medical, but there is significant social and psychiatric disability.

Histories for all somatoform disorders should reflect the same five-axial taxonomy recommended in the DSM-IV for pain evaluation:

- Anatomical region
- Organ system
- Temporal characteristics of the symptom(s) (continuous or episodic, character, pattern, setting)
- Patient's statement of severity and time since onset of symptoms
- Psychological factors (mood, anxiety, psychosis)

Other features that are of interest include:

- History of trauma and losses
- Past reaction to these events
- Psychological mindedness (i.e., expresses feelings and reactions to events, shows emotion, demonstrates empathy for others)
- Questions about the immediate family and work situation
- A thorough medical examination

- Diagnostic tests (if not already performed by the medical referring doctor) or review of records
- Neurological examination when conversion is suspected

Once the initial evaluation is completed, attention to physical symptoms should be minimized to avoid "medicalizing" the problem, and attention to psychological factors should become the dominant focus. Ideally, medical care should be handled by medical colleagues to allow the psychiatrist to maintain attention on the patient's psychological defenses, precipitating events, relationships, teaching new problem-solving and coping skills, and explaining medical issues.

CLASSIC SOMATOFORM DISORDERS

Background

The clinical distinction between somatization disorder and hypochondriasis is largely one of disease conviction. The more a patient is convinced that he or she has a disease, the more likely the patient will push for potentially harmful exploratory surgeries or dangerous treatments. A conviction of disease and insistence on treatment characterize somatization disorders. Severe somatization disorder (Briquet's syndrome) is very uncommon in older adults. This syndrome is defined by multiple complaints (at least eight) in multiple organ systems. The last large NIMH Epidemiologic Catchment Area (ECA) survey that randomly surveyed community populations in five geographic areas found a rate of somatization disorder (Briquet's) of 0% in the elderly (65+) (Meyers et al., 1984).

Hypochondriasis, the less severe state of fearing that one has a disease but being unsure, leads to help seeking but treatment refusal. Diagnostic tests are desired by the patient, but there is as much fear of harm from treatment as from having a disease, so treatment is usually rejected. In elderly populations, hypochondriasis does not spare men, as it does in younger populations. Preoccupation with symptoms mimics obsessive–compulsive disorder (OCD), depression, and psychosis (somatic delusions).

Preoccupations about health are perseverative, intrusive, and often lead to excessive emergency room visits or harm from self-treatment. Compulsive behaviors may be part of the profile; for example, calling adult children 40–50 times a day (three or four times per hour while awake) to describe a symptom. When severe, the ideation appears to be a formal thought disorder. Depressive symptoms of anergy (lack of energy), apathy (lack of interest), anhedonia (lack of pleasure), and social withdrawal are present, although often not always meeting criteria for a major depressive disorder because there are minimal mood complaints. Patients are socially withdrawn but say they would like to have more social contact if they did not feel so sick. Every complaint is attributed to a potential illness. These similarities to OCD, psychosis, and depression lead to a variety of medication trials with SSRIs, antipsychotics, and ECT.

Patients with hypochondriasis frustrate physicians because they call often, miss appointments because they feel too sick to come in, and have unlikely side effects to all medications (they often label their reactions *allergies* to medications). One physician spoke of a patient who developed a side effect if a pill came within an inch of her mouth. Somatization patients see little reason to talk about feelings because they believe their problem is purely medical. Although the patient's refusal of care keeps them safe from iatrogenic harm, there is no spontaneous recovery, and such patients remain high service users, changing doctors often and remaining miserable.

Neurobiological Explanation

The major finding underlying these syndromes is the construct of alexithymia (no words for feelings; alexithymia is not a DSM-IV personality type). Patients with alexithymia are generally concrete in their thinking; that is, they lack psychological mindedness. It appears to be a disorder of affect regulation that is the polar opposite of impulsivity or anger. Alexithymia differs from defensiveness or difficulty communicating feelings in that affected individuals literally seem to lack insight or capacity for introspection. They do not read much and do not enjoy the arts, which require abstraction and interpretation. Under overwhelming stress, these patients literally decompensate but do not acknowledge an emotional cause.

It is still unclear why alexithymic individuals cannot generate "signal anxiety" (a warning sign that something is wrong). Unlike most other personality diagnoses, the putative cause of this inability is abnormalities in areas that regulate affect; the right anterior cingulate gyrus and amygdala, deep in the temporal lobe. This finding was suggested by hypoperfusion of these areas on PET studies in alexithymic patients under stress (Taylor et al., 1999). Alexithymia is the putative basis for conversion symptoms. If a person is unable to express or show emotion, the psychological issue is said to convert to a symbolic medical symptom and is expressed physically. For example, an emotional problem will appear as a stomach ache or headache rather than an emotional complaint.

Normal versus Abnormal Behavior

Somatization patients show more abnormal personality characteristics than patients with hypochondriasis, such as more neuroticism, less extraversion, less agreeableness, and less conscientiousness on the NEO-5 scale (Extraversion, Agreeableness, Conscientiousness, Neuroticism, Openness to Experience—the original Neuroticism, Extroversion, Openness domains were expanded to five traits [Costa & McCrae, 1983; Hollifield et al., 1999]). Major depressive disorder is a common comorbidity, and suicide risk is greater in all somatoform disorders (Duberstein, 2004), but the depression is often atypical, with apathy, anergy, and other neurovegetative features as the dominant presentation. Body dysmorphic disorder (preoccupation with a defect in appearance) is rarely diagnosed in older adults, but preoccupations with appearance do exist, wherein common changes due to aging are experienced as akin to disfigurement. When body dysmorphic-like symptoms appear in older patients, they are usually labeled an adjustment disorder.

Unique Aspects of the Disorder in Elderly

Three primary psychosocial theories are particularly apropos in viewing somatoform complaints in the elderly. The first is a developmental state of hypervigilance to body changes due to increased illness risk. The second is a culturally- or cohort-based tendency to communicate emotional concerns through bodily metaphors (communication style). The third is the reappearance of narcissism and self-preoccupation as a late-life developmental theme that differs from simple hypervigilance. These three theories and their components are summarized in Table 9.1 below.

Table 9.1. Themes in Somatoform Disorders

1. Preoccupation and hypervigilance due to a real life-threatening disease.
2. Preoccupation as a communication style (e.g., cultural or learned style); somatic complaints as metaphorical communication.
3. Conversion disorder due to unacceptable internal conflict or feelings, such as a history of abuse, with some recent trigger for recurring fears.
4. Developmental task (integrity vs. despair) and resulting anxiety triggered by illness or loss.
5. Regression due to resurgence of narcissim, which is due to maladaptive thoughts about illness, biases, blind spots addressed in CBT.

Patients tend to focus their daily efforts around illness management (e.g., the majority of conversation time is spent talking about aches and pains, medications, doctor visits, and so on). Several underlying psychological factors have been suggested for somatization symptoms. In older adults, somatic preoccupations and a state of hypervigilance may represent a fear of death precipitated by illness or loss. This response pattern was predicted by Erikson's (1963) eighth stage of development, which holds that personal illness or death of a loved one triggers an introspective struggle in which one's integrity is pitted against despair. The underlying question for older adults is whether they have done everything they had planned in life, and whether they will be remembered for anything. *Integrity* is the positive outcome wherein life is felt to be meaningful. *Despair*, the opposite outcome, is related to a feeling of regret that one has failed in life and will be remembered only for one's failures. Wisdom is the ideal outcome with dogmatism, rigidity, and psychopathology at the opposite pole. Religiosity may increase as a way to transcend these existential problems (Koenig, 2004).

Somatic complaints have been viewed as a communication style for some patients. In times of stress, somatic complaints appear to be more common in patients from minority groups (U.S. Department of Health and Human Services, 2001). This pattern has been termed a meta-communication or cultural style of indirectly communicating emotional distress. The concept of an emotional problem is not alien to any culture, but how it is discussed or dealt with often differs from one culture to another. Somatic complaints based on cultural communication styles can be confronted and addressed using carefully explained and negotiated psychotherapeutic approaches.

Somatic illness can represent other underlying psychological dynamics. Symptoms of illness can be conversion phenomenon whereby a psychological conflict manifests itself as a somatic symptom. Being physically ill elicits care from others and allows one to avoid psychological awareness of an underlying and unacceptable conflict or belief. It is usually presumed that the avoided psychological issue is based in a past trauma, such as having a history of abuse or other trauma combined with a recent life situation that revives the old memories.

Another dynamic at play with somatoform disorders is the possible reappearance of narcissism and self-preoccupation—increased frailty and dependence with old age may lead to a greater focus on the self (Grotjahn, 1955). Elderly adults often appear self-centered or self-preoccupied, and communication of emotional distress may be difficult. Dependence and fearfulness when alone may be observed, with symptoms soothed by the presence of an attachment figure. Other childlike features, such as a need for transitional objects (surrounding oneself with personal possessions for security), may be heightened. Demanding, self-absorbed older adults cannot understand why others can't give them what they want or need.

It is important as a clinician to be aware that this range of somatoform symptoms probably represents regressive behavior and does not indicate a lifelong personality trait. Patients still worry about others and show empathy despite their self-preoccupations. Cognitive–behavioral therapy is often advised to reverse maladaptive thoughts about illness, biases, and blind spots, especially because a lack of psychological mindedness or introspection is thought to characterize individuals who manifest somatoform symptoms under stress.

Assessment and Diagnosis

A medical cause for symptoms should be ruled out with a physical examination and testing, which should typically be completed by the referring primary care physician (PCP). The next section in this chapter deals with syndromes in which both psychological and medical causes for symptoms are present, such as chronic pain, asthma, GI problems, fibromyalgia, or chronic fatigue syndrome. In the case of somatoform symptoms, one or more of the following is usually a sign of a classic somatoform disorder rather than a medical problem (Rubin, 2005).

- Responses are inconsistent and difficult to define (e.g., pain may feel sharp, or symptoms occur all over the body).
- Existence of *la belle indifference* (no emotion or worry is shown toward the symptom).
- If sensory loss is present, the affected dermatomes split exactly in the midline (an area of skin innervated by a single pair of peripheral nerves—right and left).
- If weakness is present, it is probably not medical if any of the following signs are present:
  - ✓ Atasia-abasia—inability to stand despite normal strength and movement when lying down or sitting.
  - ✓ Leg flexion—inability to exert pressure against resistance when sitting, despite no problems walking.
  - ✓ Hoover's sign—lack of backward pressure from the opposite leg when the patient is asked to lift his or her weak leg (no attempt to use leverage).
- Pseudoseizures are suspected if any of the following signs are present:
  - ✓ Random thrashing of all four limbs (not typical tonic-clonic movement [rapidly alternating muscular contraction and relaxation]).
  - ✓ Cyanosis (blue skin from poor oxygenation) is not present.
  - ✓ Reflexes, including papillary and corneal reflexes, remain normal.

Treatment Methods

Medications

Clinically, somatization patients must be protected against iatro-genic harm from unnecessary invasive medical procedures and medications.

When anxiety is a dominant feature of the illness, SSRIs rather than benzodiazepines have become the treatment of choice for older adults to avoid dependence, confusion, and risk of falls. Benzodiazepines such as lorazepam, at doses 2 mg/day, and supportive psycho-therapy are useful during titration of an SSRI, but should not be considered a long-term treatment. Antidepressants and atypical antipsychotics are often given off-label, but are relatively ineffective.

Psychosocial Interventions

The lack of a therapeutic alliance, which is evident from patients' doctor shopping, is the most serious barrier to effective treatment and makes expressive or behavioral therapies extremely difficult. In order to establish a working alliance, one must get patients into the office and see them on a regular schedule and frequently. An old joke states that "if psychotherapy doesn't work, prescribe more of it." This is usually meant as a criticism of psychotherapy, but in this case it leads to a patient's trust and involvement. Patients who call often must be told that their frequent phone calls mean that they need to come for sessions more often because they are seeking help. It is important to point out that they are coming because they are sick and that they should never say they are too sick to come in. Ultimately, patients who improve can be seen less often after working through the psychological fear that fewer sessions are a sign of abandonment.

Telephone sessions can be arranged in some situations but are not a covered service under Medicare. In all sessions with somatization patients, it is important to give undivided attention to them and not allow telephone calls or interruptions during the session.

The general steps to improve the therapeutic alliance can be considered "rules of engagement"—that is, factors that (1) reduce patient acting out and therapist acting out (i.e. being critical or even insulting) and (2) help create a supportive environment (holding environment) for treatment (Blazer, 1990).

Rules of Engagement:
- Patients must agree that the purpose of treatment is to try to control symptoms without medications (unless there is a clear-cut major depression or psychosis).
- Patients must agree to keep regular appointments (usually weekly).
- Patients must agree that "The worse you feel, the more you need to keep your appointment" (exceptions—patient has a temperature or is in the hospital).
- Patients agree to think about what was discussed outside of the session (and do homework when cognitive—behavioral approaches are used).
- Patients must understand that there is no substitution for coming regularly; they must see you face-to-face for all communication.
- Patients must understand why you will not accept their telephone calls between sessions, especially if they miss a session.
- Patients should still be able to call if they have a true emergency; mislabeling something an emergency when it is not should becomes a therapeutic issue.
- Prescriptions will not be refilled by telephone.

Items to emphasize during sessions are listed below.

Secondary Rules:
- A focused examination of the patient's physical complaint is needed on each visit, but medical discussions should never be the main purpose for a visit. Involve other medical specialties to perform the physical examination and laboratory testing as required.
- Do not ask leading questions. Many will say "Yes" to almost every question or say "I don't know" to please you and avoid meaningful self-disclosure.
- Be unambiguous. Use short, simple statements or questions (not compound ones).
- When inferring underlying mood and affect from nonverbal

cues, it is important to ask for feedback from the patient. For example, "You looked upset when we talked about . . ." This is a gentle form of confrontation.

- Be more transparent with feelings (modeling) than is typical with other patients. It is permissible to say "If that were me, I would feel . . ." or "I feel so sad hearing that . . ."
- Because it is important to the patient, begin each session talking about new medical issues or reviewing labs and tests, but this should not exceed 5 minutes of the session.
- Never talk about cure, talk about symptom control.
- Avoid venturing a diagnosis or prognosis.
- Do not minimize the patient's experience (never say "it is all in their head"). For example, a colleague labels pseudo-seizures (a conversion disorder) as non-epileptic seizures because the symptoms are real to the patient and his term seems less offensive.
- If patients call a lot between sessions, increase the frequency of sessions.
- Use psychiatric medications sparingly and not for off-label indications.

Psychotherapy

No controlled studies have been done on the effectiveness or duration of different therapies for somatoform disorders in older adults. Those who have shown the best response to psychotherapy are more psychologically minded and have good social supports, as summarized in Table 9.3.

Table 9.3. Psychosocial Factors Facilitating Good Prognosis for Somatoform Disorders

Insight
- Accepts concept of psychologically based symptoms.
- Insight regarding potential stressors.

Social supports
- Supportive and loving marital partner and family actively involved.

Attitude toward psychotherapy (motivation for treatment)
- Reports benefiting from prior treatment and experiences relief from talking.
- Compliant with medical treatments.
- Stays with physicians for reasonable lengths of time (gives them a chance).

Table 9.3. (continued)

Reports feeling better by the end of the first session.
Tried self-help (e.g., relaxation techniques).
Is nondefensive.
Has no obvious secondary gain (attention, sympathy, financial gain, avoidance of
    something).
Has history of being independent.
Does not withhold information (e.g., does not initially deny certain treatments
    only to say "I tried that and it made me sick" or "I'm taking that medication
    now") when something is suggested.

Source: Adapted from Rubin (2005).

It should be evident that many somatization patients who lack
insight (and lack humor) have limited social supports because of
their personalities and behaviors. Cognitive–behavioral therapy
(CBT) appears to be the most effective approach for this type of
patient because it teaches social and problem-solving skills (Clark,
2006; Allen et al., 2006; Lombardo, 2005). In CBT, patients
must often first be convinced that their complaints are related to
stress by keeping diaries of what they are doing or thinking when
symptoms begin, and learning the temporal association between
symptoms and events. Patients learn to identify stressors, plan
lifestyle changes (to avoid stressors), and practice relaxation techniques. They must often be encouraged to do "homework." New
social and individual coping skills are developed (e.g., problem-
solving steps, generalization).

As described in Chapter 7, except for universal threats to life,
which are always stressful, other issues are perceived as a threat
because of how they are appraised. When an individual believes
that something is dangerous and that he or she has no control
over it, it is stressful. Novel situations can seem stressful or excit-
ing, depending upon how one views them. Reexposure to prior
stressful conditions is stressful if the individual still feels the situation cannot be controlled. Cognitive limitations can make any
situation appear stressful because the appraisal is impaired, and
everything seems overwhelming.

The goals of treatment are actually tangential to the primary
complaint, namely to:

- Identify potential stresses that lead to symptoms.
- Learn stress reduction and participate in relaxation training.
- Learn to deal with a stressor through practice and rehearsal (mastery).
- Learn problem-solving strategies.
- Learn to self-monitor and manage medical aspects of the disease (increase a sense of control).
- Reestablish a positive support network that reinforces the individual's attempts at autonomy and does not create dependence.

Successfully achieving these goals decreases the sense of threat and creates a sense of understanding and control of the situation. Cognitive–behavioral therapy seems best suited for these limited goals.

When patients show some insight and are more psychologically minded about underlying repressed conflicts, "exploratory" psychodynamic treatment models may be effective, as suggested in older treatment models. If the interpretation is accepted, the patient will become more open and show an increase in relevant associated memories.

Family or couple interventions are sometimes needed to restore support networks and reduce overt interpersonal conflicts. Self-help groups or supportive group therapies are often helpful in modeling behaviors.

Although encouraging autonomy is common, there are a few situations in which pushing for it or for insight is not beneficial. At times accepting a patient's need for dependence and gratifying it may eliminate somatic complaints, such as a frail patient in a nursing home setting.

GENERAL MEDICAL CONDITION WITH OR WITHOUT PSYCHOLOGICAL FACTORS

This type of psychosomatic illness is listed in the DMS-IV-TR as "Psychological Factors Affecting Medical Conditions" (316). It is defined by the presence of one or more specific psychological or behavioral factors that adversely affect a general medical condition. The relationship is bidirectional: Psychiatric factors can worsen or cause a medical condition such as asthma, peptic ulcers, ulcerative colitis, fibromyalgia, chronic fatigue, and pain. Medical problems can worsen or cause psychiatric problems (i.e., hypothyroidism causing depression, or the effects of a stroke, cardiovascular disease, interferon, renal disease, or occult effects of cancer causing depression). This effect of medical illness on depression is thought to go beyond a simple adjustment reaction because it occurs in the absence of a disability, medical instability, or overt worries or concern about the disease.

Background

The classic list of psychosomatic illnesses are asthma, hypertension, rheumatoid arthritis, ulcerative colitis, thyrotoxicosis, neurodermatitis, and peptic ulcer disease (Alexander, French & Pollock, 1968). Complaints of excess pain and worsening cardiac symptoms (angina, chest pain) have traditionally been added to this spectrum. These are conditions that have been associated with increased risk of occurrence at times of stress. Fibromyalgia and chronic fatigue syndrome (CFS) are new to this list, the result of recent genetic findings, many involving autoimmune pathways, which will be described in more detail in the next section (Vernon & Reeves, 2006; Whistler, Taylor, Kraddock, et al., 2006). These two conditions presumably occur because of a genetic vulnerability that causes an abnormal stress response.

Colds during times of stress, delayed recovery from illness, and increased risk of hypertension, angina, myocardial infarctions or strokes under stress are additional common examples of psychosomatic illnesses. Responses after a disaster also exemplify this effect, as seen in older adults following Hurricane Katrina in 2005, where there was not only a marked increase in major depression and anxiety, but also a worsening or onset of a host of diseases such as hypertension, heart disease, and diabetes (Weisler & Barbee, 2006).

The reverse issue—that is, medical conditions causing depression—is also well established. Estimates of the prevalence of major depression in patients with comorbid medical illness range from 4% to 75% (Evans, Charney, Lewis, et al., 2005).

The diseases that show higher rates of depression as a comorbidity are cardiac disease, cerbrovascular disease, Alzheimer's disease, Parkinson's disease, epilepsy, diabetes, cancer, chronic pain states, and HIV/AIDS. The highest rates appear to occur in Parkinson's patients (4% to 75%), poorly controlled epilepsy (20% to 55%), and chronic pain states (30% to 45%); intermediate rates were associated with cardiac disease and cancer (17% to 29%); and lowest rates occur in controlled chronic disorders. The risk of developing major depression with cardiac disease is 1.64 times greater for patients than for controls (Evans, Charney, Lewis, et al., 2005).

Neurobiological Explanation

Dysfunction in the HPA axis has been postulated as a major mediating factor in psychosomatic illness for over 60 years (Selye, 1956, 1978). This dysfunction is also a hypothetical mediator of increased rates of depression and anxiety with illness, particularly in endocrinopathies, cerebral ischemia (especially in subcortical regions), and neurodegenerative processes (Evans, Charney, Lewis, et al., 2005). The HPA axis modulates the limbic system and is associated with mood and other psychiatric symptomatology as well as disease symptoms. Changes in the HPA axis also involve other stress-related changes in catecholamines, amino acids, and neuropeptides.

HPA axis dysfunction is the basis of the dexamethasone test. Under usual conditions cortisol levels show a diurnal variation, low at night and high in the morning. One mg of dexamethasone is given at 11:00 PM to suppress the surge of cortisol at 8:00 AM the next morning. An abnormal finding is seen in depression, AD, chronic stress, and a variety of disorders. Instead of extremely low cortisol levels in the AM following dexamethasone administration, the AM cortisol levels remain in the high to normal range (nonsuppressed). In PTSD and bipolar disorders, in particular, the diurnal variation in cortisol secretion is also no longer suppressed and constantly remains at the high end of the normal range. In older adults, the relatively constant high cortisol stimulation may lead to cognitive dysfunction and even cortical atrophy (Egeland, Lund, Landro, et al., 2005; Magri, Cravello, Barli, et al., 2006;

Watson, Thompson, Ritchie, et al., 2006). In normally functioning older adults, higher mean cortisol levels are associated with poorer declarative memory and executive function (Li, Cherrier, Tsuang, et al., 2006)

A large body of scientific studies have elucidated the actions of hormones such as cortisol on membrane receptors (on the cell surface) and nuclear receptors (in the cell itself). Membrane receptors include G-protein coupled receptors (GPCR), tyrosine kinase receptors (where growth hormone acts), cytokine receptors, and serine kinase receptors. Over a hundred small molecules, such as cortisol, thyroid hormone, and gonadotropins (sex hormones) comprise the nuclear receptors that increase or decrease gene transcription (Jameson, 2001).

Genes that code for the proteins involved in autoimmune pathways have been targeted for study. Candidate genes are those that code for proteins and are critical in the biological pathways underlying the disease in question. If an association is confirmed, "designer medications" that might restore function in these pathways may be tested as potential treatments. The complex interaction that controls the immune response or hyper-response can be reviewed in related chapters of Kaplan and Sadock's *Comprehensive Textbook of Psychiatry* (Sadock & Sadock, 2004) and Harrison's *Principles of Internal Medicine* (Kasper, Braunwald, Fauci, et al., 2005).

A series of papers in the March 2006 issue of *Pharmacogenomics* from the Witchita CFS (chronic fatigue syndrome) Project determined the existence of two differently expressed gene lists, one for CFS and the other for depression (Witkowski, 2006). Fifty percent of the associated genes were expected and fit pathways of cytokine-cytokine receptor interaction and neuroreaction, but 50% were unexpected and of unknown cause (Vernon & Reeves, 2006). The papers addressed new statistical approaches to the same data. In regard to psychosomatic illnesses in general, genetic profiling may ultimately reduce the uncertainty of our current diagnostic approaches and allow for specific treatments based on specific genetic abnormalities. Psychiatric diseases with a known genetic link are included in the OMIM (Online Mendelian Inheritance in Man, 2006), developed for the National Center for Biotechnology Information.

Normal Versus Abnormal Behavior

Although rarely presented in this way, a key concept in psychosomatic illness lies in understanding and managing "allostatic load." *Allostatis* refers to the ability to maintain stability in the face of variable situations (Stewart, 2006). This is different from *homeostasis*, which refers to the maintenance of stability in an unchanging set of circumstances. One assumes that social situations and life in general are never static. Patients must learn to accept change.

The problem for patients with psychosomatic diseases is the inability to change appropriately to changing conditions. Asthma is just one example of a condition for which there are abundant objective data that psychological factors interact with the asthmatic diathesis to worsen or ameliorate the disease process. This interaction occurs in possibly half the patients studied (McFadden, 2001). Although no single pheonotype defines asthma, genes from multiple chromosomal regions have been mapped that explain the fundamental mechanisms underlying the illness. It is assumed that subacute inflammation, which is partly an autoimmune process, may be present. High total serum immunoglobin-E (IgE) levels and atopy have been related to chromosomes 5q, 11q, and 12q (hereditary predisposition to hypersensitivity), which have been associated with asthma. Histamine, bradykinin, leukotrines, platelet-activating factor, and prostaglandins are all peptides and lipids that have been linked to heightened airway reactivity (bronchial constriction), which are part of the autoimmune pathway and are, in turn, controlled by emotional factors.

A historical aspect of psychosomatic illness that deserves mention is the concept of *organ specificity*. This pre-genetic concept was used to explain why some people are vulnerable and can't adapt to changing conditions. It was believed that the reason some people developed asthma, others heart attacks, and others ulcers when faced with stress was due to "zonal fixation" on an organ system, which reflected an underlying, symbolic area of psychosocial conflict. This belief was evident in many psychoanalytically-oriented writings of the 1960s including Eric Erikson's theory of the eight stages of development (1963). "Trust versus mistrust" characterized an oral fixation (putting everything into the mouth or rejecting it); "autonomy versus shame and doubt" characterized an anal fixation (bowel control); and so forth. The contemporary version of this argument is the concept of an environment-gene interaction whereby genes may not only make individuals vulnerable to certain illnesses, but may draw people into situations and relationships that reinforce the expression of their genetic predispositions.

It is interesting that this organ fixation theory was put to the test in a unique study conducted by the Chicago Psychoanalytic Institute, which was alluded to earlier (Alexander, French & Pollock, 1968). In this study, psychoanalysts interviewed patients who had traditional psychosomatic illnesses (asthma, hypertension, rheumatoid arthritis, ulcerative colitis, thyrotoxicosis, neurodermatitis, and peptic ulcer disease), but only took developmental histories. Internists listened to audiotapes of the interviews to be sure they could not make a medical diagnosis based on what the patients revealed. The psychoanalysts made the most likely medical diagnosis (of the options above) based solely on personality and developmental histories, postulating that an earlier, central psychological conflict would lead to a breakdown in the individual's primary defenses for that organ (Alexander, French & Pollack, 1968). The psychoanalysts' diagnoses were often correct.

Unique Aspects of the Disorder in Elderly

Although not entirely restricted to older adults, persistent pain is an extremely common complaint. Persistent pain syndromes commonly occur in primary care patients in all cultures, and 50% of patients with persistent pain syndromes do not admit to any improvement after one year (Gureje, Simon, & Von Korff, 2001). In the older population, pain complaints are almost always associated with a general medical condition (307.89), and psychological factors play an important role in determining the onset, severity, exacerbation, or persistence of pain.

Pain circuits are closely tied to pathways that regulate mood and cognition. Primary afferent nocioreceptors (pain receptors that send information to the brain) are comprised of several categories of nerve fibers (Ab, Ad, and unmyelinated C fiber axons) that end in the midbrain, thalamus, and sensory cortex. Many hormones, peptides (building blocks for proteins), and lipids (fats) are produced and released throughout the body and brain to mediate pain perception, either when pain occurs or when it is anticipated. These agents include prostaglandins, prostacyclin, bradykinin, histamine, and serotonin. An enzyme that creates prostaglandins and increases the pain response is COX-2 (cyclooxygenase-2; Fields & Martin, 2000). Medicines that block COX-2, like celicoxib, act differently than older pain medications and have become a new generation of pain medications. Psychotherapy helps to build a sense of control over pain (coping or altered appraisal of the situation), and reduces pain complaints while minimizing the need for medication.

Assessment and Diagnosis

In assessing psychological influences on medical conditions, a traditional psychiatric interview is needed. Personality trait testing such as the 16PF or MMPI are usually not required. Special attention should be placed on temporal relationships between perceived stress or timing of illness to life events, interpersonal difficulties, and the presence of depression.

One measure developed for depression screening in a general office setting is the PRIME-MD (Primary Care Evaluation of Mental Disorders, Patient Health Questionnaire; Spitzer, Kroenke, & Williams, 1999). This self-report questionnaire can be completed in the waiting room and is easily scored. The periodic application of the PRIME-MD is advisable if time does not permit longer face-to-face interviews during routine psychiatric visits.

The psychiatrist should pay particular attention to and identify early substance abuse, delirium, dementia, affective disorders, anxiety disorders, and suicidal ideation. He or she should also evaluate the adequacy of the patient's coping, family support, and state of worry precipitated by chronic illness.

Chronic fatigue syndrome (CFS) occurs frequently in the elderly, but is underdiagnosed. The diagnostic criteria require six months of duration with medical causes excluded by clinical diagnosis and four or more of the following symptoms: substantial impairment in short-term memory or concentration; sore throat or tender lymph nodes; muscle pain; multijoint pain without swelling or redness; headaches of a new type, pattern, or severity; unrefreshing sleep; and post-exertional malaise lasting more than 24 hours (Centers for Disease Control, 2006).

A long list of medical diseases and medications that cause psychiatric symptoms that require special attention. Cognitive change (delirium, confusion, sedation) related to medication or illness is the most common abnormality. However, depression, psychosis, and agitation also occur frequently. The disorders are classified under several different categories in the DSM-IV-TR, including psychiatric problems due to a general medical condition (e.g., endocrinopathies, 293.8x; dementia with behavior disturbance, 290.4x and 294.11; delirium, 293.0; and substance-induced disorders, 291.0–292.9). Table 9.4 summarizes the typical medical conditions that cause psychiatric symptoms in older adults.

Table 9.4. Typical Medical Conditions Causing Psychiatric Symptoms in Older Adults

DISEASE	COMMON ASSOCIATED PSYCHIATRIC SYMPTOMS
Medications (adverse effects)	"Subacute delirium" (concentration problems
Anticholinergic effects	and mild cognitive impairment), insomnia,
Steroids	sedation, depression, psychosis, anxiety
Narcotics	
Chemotherapies	
Interferon α & β	Depression
Substance Abuse & Withdrawal (usually alcohol for this age group)	
Hypothyroidism	Depression, fatigue, occasionally psychosis (20% may show symptoms)
Hyperthyroidism	Agitation, depression, psychosis
Hyperparathyrodism	Fatigue, depression, irritability
Diabetes	Anxiety, depression, confusion, agitation
Hypertension	Anxiety
	Bizarre behavior
Seizure Disorder (partial complex)	Aggression, psychosis, depression
Dementias (AD is most common, Parkinson's)	

Table 9.4. (continued)

Anemia	Fatigue, restless leg syndrome, confusion
Uremia	Agitation, psychosis, confusion
Hepatic insufficiency	Agitation, psychosis, confusion
Cerebrovascular accidents (CVA)	Varies with the lesion; depression is most common with anterior dominant hemisphere strokes (left anterior and middle cerebral artery distribution)
Subcortical ischemic changes	Depression
Delirium	Prodromal features for delirium include restlessness, anxiety, irritability, and sleep disturbance

Treatment Methods

Medications

Several studies using SSRIs in medically ill populations have shown them to be safe and effective. Use of SSRIs is advised as the initial treatment, according to a consensus conference of experts addressing the medical comorbidity in patients with mood disorders in 2002 (Evans et al., 2005). As with all major depressive disorders, ECT can be considered after two adequate antidepressant trials because it may be safer than augmentation strategies with medications, or may be necessary for psychiatric emergency situations such as suicidal risk or endangerment to self due to severe anorexia.

Treatment of pain related to a medical disorder requires special comment. Medications are still a mainstay of pain management, but their use may be reduced when psychological considerations are addressed. The World Health Organization analgesic ladder (Lederberg & Joshi, 2005) describes management with a nonopioid analgesic first (nonsteroidal anti-inflammatory drugs [NSAIDs] or acetaminophen) with or without an adjuvant such as a psychotropic (TCA, neuroleptic, anxiolytic [e.g., lorazepam], or anticonvulsant [e.g., gabapentin]). An opioid may be added for mild to moderate pain if pain persists or increases. Somnolence may require a stimulant such methylphenidate (Ritalin, Concerta) or modafinil (Provigil). Medications should be given on a by-the-clock administration with rescue doses for break-through pain. This protocol varies from the usual as-needed dosing approach. Periodic monitoring of complete blood count (CBC) and comprehensive metabolic panel (CMP) is needed to avoid a bleeding diathesis or hepatic or renal dysfunction.

Psychosocial Interventions

Unlike patients with psychiatric somatization disorders, many patients with general medical conditions welcome the opportunity to discuss hidden emotions and gain insight. One caveat, though, is that psychosomatic patients often accept treatment better if the psychiatrist is part of the treatment team and can see them in their familiar medical setting. In hospital, institution, or clinic setting, the psychiatrist can participate in rounds or team meetings to discuss problems and educate nonpsychiatric physicians about associated psychiatric themes. Assistance with family problems is often important.

A goal of psychiatric interventions is to "empower the patient," to give the patient a sense of control over the illness. David Spiegel, who was part of a group from Stanford who described physiological effects of psychosocial interventions, summarized the psychological approach through the acronym FACES (Moran, 2004; Giese-Davis et al., 2006):

F Face rather than flee (in reference to facing the
   stressful situation)
A Alter your view of the world
C Cope actively, not passively (learn problem
   solving)
E Express emotion
S Seek social support

Many of the guidelines for treating somatization patients apply to patients who have general medical conditions with psychological features. Spiritual counsel may help, and allaying unrealistic fears through active/empathic listening helps. Many of the general fears are fear of suffering, fear of isolation or abandonment, or fear of being a burden on others. Treatment generally requires long-term maintenance with antidepressant medication and supportive therapy. Cognitive–behavioral therapy has been the most widely studied approach, but other modalities should not be excluded if they better suit the patient's needs. These modalities are discussed in the next chapter.

SUMMARY

Somatoform disorders are divided into two types: (1) classic somatoform disorders such as hypochondriasis and somatization disorder, and (2) a general medical condition with or without psychological features (classic psychosomatic illness), such as pain syndromes, asthma, stress-related illness, chronic fatigue syndrome, and fibromyalgia. Hypochondriasis is the classic somatoform disorder seen in the elderly, where patients show fear that they have an illness, seek doctor appointments, but refuse to accept medications or invasive treatment. Classic somatoform patients have difficulty expressing emotion, which may be why emotional problems are symbolically converted into physical complaints, as this is the only way they can express distress. Cognitive–behavioral therapy appears to be the most effective treatment approach. Classic psychosomatic illness, on the other hand, may have strong neurobiological underpinnings. Genetically susceptible individuals develop real medical problems or symptoms when under stress. Biological treatments do not yet exist—other than antidepressants for the high rates of depression and anxiety that accompany these disorders—although they may be possible in the future as more is understood about underlying gene-environment interactions and neuronal processes.

10

PSYCHOTHERAPY WITH OLDER ADULTS

Chronological age is not a barrier to treatment. As one geriatric psychiatrist said, "Older patients who enter treatment are often more motivated to change. This is their last chance to do so." As with other patients, the challenge of doing psychotherapy with older adults is to select the best model or technique for individuals and their problems and establish a working alliance. The selection is partially based on the type of problem that a particular method was designed to address, but also involves an assessed degree of patient motivation, psychological mindedness, and cognitive abilities. Many therapists claim an "eclectic approach," meaning that they adhere to common features shared by most psychotherapies rather than a particular school of treatment. These common features include (1) an emotionally charged confiding relationship with a helping person; (2) a safe setting; (3) a rational conceptual scheme that provides an explanation of the patient's behavior and a procedure for resolving it; and (4) belief that the procedure will help. These features all require a working alliance as an essential starting point in psychotherapy. Successful therapist characteristics are nonpossessive warmth, accurate empathy, therapeutic genuineness, and respect (Patterson, 2000). The main schools of therapy listed in the DSM-IV-TR are listed in Table 10.1.

Studies confirm the efficacy of psychotherapy with older adults (Sadavoy & Lazarus, 2004), and the same recommendation applies to this population that is given for younger populations: that combined psychotherapy and pharmacotherapy are better than either alone for major psychiatric disorders. Although no theoretical school of psychotherapy has evolved specifically for geriatric patients, work with this population seems very different to the nonspecialist. But keep in mind that the goal of therapy for all populations, from a developmental perspective, is to help people through a temporary obstacle in their own course of life, and not to push for some abstract ideal outcome. Goal-setting should be done early in the course of treatment.

Table 10.1. Types of Psychotherapy

I. RECONSTRUCTIVE

A. Psychoanalysis—Sigmund Freud
B. Neo-Freudian modifications of psychoanalysis
   1. Active analytic techniques—Sandor Ferenczi, Wilhelm Stekel, the Chicago school (especially Franz Alexander and Thomas French)
   2. Analytic psychology—Carl Jung
   3. Character analysis, orgone therapy—Wilhelm Reich
   5. Ego psychology—Rudolph Loewenstein
   8. Object relations—Otto Kernberg
   9. Self psychology—Heinz Kohut
   10. Existential analysis—Ludwig Binswanger
   11. Holistic analysis—Karen Horney
   12. Individual psychology—Alfred Adler
   13. Transactional analysis—Eric Berne
   14. Washington cultural school—Harry Stack Sullivan, Erich Fromm, Clara Thompson
   15. Will therapy—Otto Rank
C. Group approaches
   1. Orthodox psychoanalytic—S. R. Slavson
   2. Psychodrama—J. L. Moreno
   3. Psychoanalysis in groups—Alexander Wolf
   4. Valence systems—W. R. Bion

II. REEDUCATIVE AND SUPPORTIVE, INDIVIDUAL AND GROUP

A. Client-centered (nondirective)—Carl Rogers
B. Conditioning, behavior therapy, behavior modification
   1. Aversion therapy—N. V. Kantorovich
   2. Behaviorism—John B. Watson
   3. Classical conditioning—Ivan Pavlov
   4. Operant conditioning—B. F. Skinner
   5. Sexual counseling—William Masters, Virginia Johnson
   6. Systematic desensitization—Joseph Wolpe
C. Cognitive–behavior therapy—Aaron Beck
D. Family therapy—Nathan Ackerman
E. Gestalt—Wolfgang Köhler, Kurt Lewin, Fritz Perls

Table 10.1. (continued)

F. Logotherapy—Viktor Frankl
G. Psychobiology (distributive analysis and synthesis)—Adolf Meyer
H. Zen (satori)—Alan Watts

Source: Adapted from American Psychiatric Association (2000; omitting treatments specific for children).

WHAT IS DIFFERENT ABOUT PSYCHOTHERAPY WITH OLDER ADULTS?

Older adults, like younger patients, respond to psychotherapy and require different approaches based on personality, cognitive function, motivation, and the nature of the problem. However, common themes differ for elderly compared to younger patients. Historically, psychoanalytically oriented psychotherapy dominated late-life psychotherapy and led to the definition of core themes of dependence, role change, fear of death, narcissistic issues (leaving a legacy, being remembered), and reemergence of unfulfilled needs (Nemiroff & Colarusso, 1985). It became common to conceptualize treatment from a grief and mourning perspective. Even illness was viewed as the loss of one's physical abilities. Currently, cognitive–behavioral therapy (social skills training, cognitive restructuring of maladaptive thoughts) and behavioral therapy for pathological behaviors in dementia have become more popular than psychodynamic approaches, because of structured methods that seem easier to teach and understand.

Techniques must often be modified to accommodate the following issues:

- Sensory impairment (communication problems)
- Cognitive impairment
- Different concerns than younger adults (core themes)
- Education and cultural barriers:
  - ✓ Many older adults are foreign born
  - ✓ Many have less than a high school education
  - ✓ Many lack "health-care literacy"—may be a factor causing stigma or reverse bias

- Slower pace of sessions, longer time needed
- Stigma and resistance by the patient and its reverse of countertransference or bias by the therapist

Holding Environment

The notion of a "holding environment" in psychoanalysis is a stable setting wherein one feels safe to explore emotions and finds an empathic figure with whom to work. For the elderly, this usually means that discussion of major life changes, like relocation, should be initially avoided in order to first secure a safe and strong therapeutic rapport. If a patient wants to move, discussion of this possibility should occur after treatment has been in progress for some time. If this holding environment is achieved in psychoanalysis, appointments should be hard to forget because they are regularly scheduled and viewed by the patient as a stable, constant event.

Missing an appointment and then calling to talk, arriving late, or trying to extend an appointment time by bringing something up at the end of the session must all be addressed as disruptions of the holding environment, as in any therapy. It is important to establish clear boundaries about frequency of sessions and session duration, and insist that patients come in more often if they feel the need to call.

Eventually, creating expectability and stability in the environment will carry over into the patient's daily life as they begin to seek regular contact with family, resolve disputes early, and re-establish a stable support network in lieu of devaluing and complaining.

Countertransference

Countertransference is no longer viewed as the therapist's projection of his or her own repressed feelings or reactions onto the patient. It is more generally thought to be any negative feeling directed toward the patient. In our context of geriatric psychiatry, negative feelings might be referred to as "ageism," but also appear as a lack of empathy for the older person—a "generation gap." In all cases it represents unjustified negative stereotypes and marginalization of older adults. Older patients often tell the joke about when they told their doctor that their left knee hurt. The doctor said, "What do you expect? You're 90 years old!" Their reply was, "I know Doc, but my right knee is 90 too, and it doesn't hurt!" Butler and Lewis (1977) suggested that unjustified therapeutic nihilism toward older patients was related to (1) stimulation of the therapist's fears about aging, (2) stimulation of the therapist's own parental conflicts (traditional countertransference), (3) anticipated therapeutic impotence, (4) wish to avoid "wasting time," (5) fears the patient may die, and (6) embarrassment about colleagues' negative comments.

Refusing to accept Medicare because it does not pay well while accepting other insurances may also represent a countertransference issue, given that Medicare often pays better than many insurance or managed care companies.

The main point is that the therapist has to take special care not to infantilize the older person, to attend to nonverbal cues and latent meanings when communication barriers exist, and to examine his or her potential countertransference bias if unable to work well with this population. Although taking notes during a session is becoming commonplace, this may not be best with elderly patients for whom nonverbal communication must be more closely observed.

Are Motives and Feelings Conceptualized Differently?

The most widely accepted views of the drives and motives underlying human behavior have origins from Abraham Maslow's Hierarchy of Needs (1943), David McClelland's ideas of n-achievement, n-power, n-affiliation (McClelland, 1975; McClelland, Atkinson, Clark & Lowell, 1953), and Sigmund Freud's drive theory (1986). These drives and motives include:

- Physiological needs (food, housing, comfort, sex)
- Safety needs
- Need for belonging (need for affiliation and social connection)
- Esteem needs (narcissistic needs)
- Need for autonomy/mastery/competence
- Cognitive-based generativity needs (need for achievement, need to leave a legacy or be remembered)

- Need for power/control
- Aesthetic needs
- Spiritual needs

The drive to discover the meaning of life and the gratification or frustration of reaching that achievement directs our life satisfaction, and should influence the approach to therapeutic treatment. Some of the related trends seen in late life are:

- Heightened importance of physiological and safety needs
- Increased need for intimacy (fewer relationships but deeper meaning)
- Less need for power or control over others (a mellowing)
- Increased need for generativity (meaning to one's life)
- Less need for mastery or achievement (more accepting, less rigid)
- Greater spirituality
- Rise in narcissism for those with dementia
- Less conflict and more focus on loss and intimacy issues

These trends in motives and values do tend to lead to the stereotypical *wise sage*—the mature individual who is slow to anger, has the capacity for close relationships, shows good judgment of people, can trust without being manipulated, is ethical and not rigid or dogmatic about beliefs, is able to look at the worst situation with a sense of humor, maintains a firm sense about his or her own beliefs and identity, is effective in problem solving, and can balance personal needs with the needs of others. However, many people need help achieving this state.

In treatment, older adults may appear non-introspective because of their externalized focus and expansiveness. They may see relationships between everything, or think they said or did something because of implicit associations in their minds. They often ask the therapist about personal information and may exaggerate their concern for others to avoid self-disclosure. These habits reflect the meaning they currently have for life—a need for intimacy but also a certain amount of ambivalence—and are not necessarily indicative of displacement.

Viewing behavior from this vantage point, there are two general approaches that the therapist should take. The first is to be more transparent with older patients than with other patients, even in psychodynamic psychotherapy. Transparency means sharing your feelings as a therapist, like being appreciative or upset by something that they said, and even sharing some personal information if asked, like how many children you have or what part of the city you live in. Boundary violations are not as much of a risk with older patients, unless the therapist begins to share negative information or makes the patient feel as if the tables have been turned and they're the therapist. Transparency is used to maintain a positive alliance and not insult the patient by withholding.

The second approach the therapist should take is contextualization. Assume everything a patient does is intelligible and adaptive from the patient's point of view. One must try to understand how even the most bizarre action or poor judgment made sense to the patient.

USEFUL PSYCHOANALYTIC CONSTRUCTS

From a psychodynamic perspective, there are six developmental lines: (1) psychosexual maturation, (2) drive-taming processes (handling aggression), (3) object relation formation (ability to form "deep relationships," including empathy), (4) adaptive functioning (perception, cognition, and skills), (5) defensive functioning (hierarchy of defenses from denial to intellectualization to humor), and (6) identify formation (superego, healthy narcissism) (Blank & Blank, 1979).

With the elderly, one usually thinks of their problems as indicating a regression in one or two lines of development, rather than a developmental arrest, which is often seen in younger patients. The developmental lines that have regressed are the points of conflict that need attention. It is important to speculate on the reason for regression in treatment. Problems may be due to a revival of long hidden issues that have resurfaced because of life experiences. An example is a patient with mild cognitive impairment who cannot handle aggression as readily as he could when he was younger and is having significant problems maintaining relationships due to longstanding conflicts over authority and control. Understanding that this is a repetition of an old problem allows the therapist to help the patient recognize a pattern to the behavior and generalize from solutions found by working through transference reactions with the therapist. The use of transference to bring about change means that the patient views the therapist as a conflictual figure from their past (e.g., a parent, if that was the problem). The therapist confronts and interprets this distorted view and shows the impact it is having in the session. The patient learns from the experience to stop further repetition. This approach could be as useful as it is with younger patients if applied correctly.

Therapeutic Concerns in Working with Older Adults

Neugarten (1979) described the importance of expectability; "off-synch" experiences are more likely to cause anxiety and emotional disturbance than expected changes. For example, the loss of a child is more stressful than the loss of a spouse to an older person, even when considering long years of attachment to the spouse. Children are supposed to outlive their parents. This reality implies that normal grief and mourning usually occur in the loss of a spouse (it was inevitable and one must move on), but in the loss of a child it lingers on.

To maintain continuity of care for the very frail elder, some patients may need planned telephone sessions instead of office visits. Individual psychotherapy can also be effective with sessions only once or twice per month if the patient is highly motivated and processes material between visits. Intensive outpatient programs (IOPs) that meet two to three times per week, for a half day, are another alternative that also allows multidisciplinary care and socialization.

Addressing Barriers to Treatment

Hearing loss with age, called *presbyacousia*, is mainly caused by sensorineural damage to the hair cells of the organ of Corti, causing loss of high-frequency tones (cannot hear consonants, making speech unintelligible; < 30% word recognition). This deterioration is usually due to chronic noise exposure throughout life, but has also been associated with medications such as salicylates or loop diuretics for hypertension. Hearing aids should be used but sometimes do not help because the hair cells that are the primary sensors are dysfunctional. Furthermore, patients often refuse to use hearing aids due to discomfort. Cochlear implants to simulate an auditory signal rather than amplify sounds are available but rarely applied with older adults. Sign language and lip reading are usually too difficult for older adults to learn, partly due to difficulty learning a second language as well as visual problems due to cataracts (lens opacities) and macular degeneration (excessive pigmentation over the visual cells).

The best assistance for presbyacousia is not talking louder but talking in lower tones, talking more slowly, and exaggerating tonal inflection of each syllable to make it distinct without hearing high-pitched consonants. Communication via a computer screen is also useful, although large print is usually needed. For an average typist (50 words/minute), typing is about one-third as fast as normal speech.

For the initial evaluation, scales such as the Symptom Checklist–90 (SCL-90) can be used if speech or hearing limit communication. Patients can read and respond to each question if they can see and have sufficient education.

SPECIFIC THERAPIES USED WITH OLDER ADULTS

The cases below demonstrate how similar problems with depression require markedly different therapeutic approaches.

CASE EXAMPLES

Mrs. J is a 76-year-old widow who entered treatment for depression. The precipitating event was the arrest (for tax evasion) of her 37-year-old unmarried son and her main support. The patient was 39 years old before she had her first child. She viewed her son's birth as a miracle and idealized him throughout his life. Rather than thoughts of anger or disappointment in her son, she focused blame on how harsh the IRS was towards him. The patient was a religious woman who was raised in a small town with a minister as a father. She was a stay-at-home mother her whole life who doted on her family. She was a penultimate volunteer, reader, and lover of the arts.

Her current life had become fairly isolated with her closest friends having moved away or fallen ill.

Commentary: Mrs. J had her world view of ethics, beliefs about her son, and her identity as a good mother challenged by this arrest incident. Because finding meaning in life may have heightened importance as one ages, her sense of integrity was shaken. Denial and projection of blame onto the IRS were her methods of coping. One would expect that she has the capacity for introspection and psychological mindedness based on her past interests. A short-term, insight-oriented therapeutic approach might be most effective.

Mrs. K is a 60-year-old divorced woman with three children. She is an anxious woman who presented with depression, suicidal ideation, and a wish to escape her daily hassles. The precipitating event was the near-death beating suffered by her only son. He had been in prison for the past 10 years, and just days before his scheduled release the beating occurred. She also talked about her middle daughter only visiting when she needs money, and her youngest daughter being rebellious and on drugs. The patient tends to deal with problems by avoidance and does not tell her family any of the criticisms she relays to doctors. She has been psychiatrically hospitalized several times for nervous breakdowns. The patient came from a lower socioeconomic class and a religious family. She was divorced when the children were young and raised them as a single mother. Her family criticizes her for being simultaneously volatile and not speaking her mind. She has said she wants to move to a different city and never see her family again.

Commentary: Mrs. K tried very hard to make a stable life for herself, finishing high school, working steadily in a clerical position, and wanting to create a better life for her children. She lacks insight and uses immature defenses of denial and projection. Given her past history, she differs from the case above in showing fragility and no evidence of insight or psychological mindedness. The patient seems to lack effective coping or problem solving skills. She might do best with a CBT approach to help her identify problems earlier, plan solutions, learn alternative coping and problem solving skills, and learn relaxation methods.

Reminiscence Therapy (Noninterpretive Model)

The value of reminiscence for elderly was first pointed out by Butler (1963). This approach has been described as a therapeutic technique and involves anamnestic recall (remembrance of the past) and free association without interpretation. It is based on the belief that transitions between life stages are dealt with by a life review. The process is a means of communication, allows one to leave behind a legacy of memories and family knowledge, allows a displaced expression of emotion, helps deal with personal loss, and may help reintegrate the personality by "taking stock" of one's lessons from life. Reminiscence therapy can be done through semistructured storytelling about different epochs of life, either individually or in groups. Reminiscence may be assisted by aids such as videos, pictures, and life story books. The value has been especially notable in early dementia as a means to reduce agitation and improve mood and cognition. It is usually done weekly, and improvement is seen within 4–6 weeks (Cochrane Collaboration Reviews, 2005; Cohen & Taylor, 1998; Woods et al., 2006).

Psychoanalytic Psychotherapy (Interpretive Model)

Freud thought that elderly people are more prone to ramble and have so many memories and so much material to present that it would take forever to analyze. At the turn of the 20th century the "elderly" were people in their 40s. Like any scientist, Freud probably thought it best to study people who showed fewer variables, such as younger patients. Freud's early warning, however, had the negative aspect of deterring the use of psychoanalytic psychotherapy with older adults for decades. The relative contraindications to psychoanalysis are poor patient motivation, cognitive impairment, poor psychological mindedness, or more circumscribed issues that are better helped by CBT. If indicated, psychoanalytically oriented psychotherapy is usually done one to two times per week, face to face, for over 6 months.

CASE EXAMPLE

Mrs. X is a 72-year-old woman who has cared for her 95-year-old mother who was recently placed in a nursing home for medical reasons. Mrs. X has felt dominated by her mother throughout life but has had unacceptable (to her) feelings of rage and resentment, followed by guilt, engendered by her mother's increasing demands in this new setting. Mrs. X feels she cannot do anything she wants to do and is unappreciated. Her current problem clearly stems from longstanding conflicts and suppressed memories that have been revived. She sought a traditional psychoanalysis at the age of 72 because of the longstanding nature of her conflicts with her mother.

Several techniques may be needed to help perform psychoanalytically-oriented therapy with the elderly. The focusing technique (Gendlin, 1981) is a method of linking somatic symptoms with underlying feelings. It uses a variety of approaches including imagery, labeling somatic sensations with affective terms ("handles"), and meditation. A second technique is to have a structured approach to dream work. One such approach is the RISC model (Cartwright, 1993), which stands for *r*ecognize when a dream is not going well, *i*dentify what is frightening, *s*top the dream, and *c*hange the action to a positive outcome. These steps are applied to the retelling of the dream, whereby the outcome can be altered. Another technique is to use a modified TAT approach (thematic apperception test) in which the older adult's story serves as a way to tap into who the people in the story are, what they are thinking and feeling, what they want to happen, what actually happened, how each person in the story feels about what happened, and what will happen next. For poorly educated older adults it may be necessary to make the story nontechnical, almost folksy.

Several short-term psychoanalytically-oriented therapies have evolved with limited goals, although none has been studied specifically in older adults.

Cognitive Therapy

Maladaptive thoughts are often thought to underlie psychiatric disorders, although the thoughts are not bizarre or psychotic.

Maladaptive depressive thoughts involve beliefs of being deficient, helpless, unlovable, guilt ridden (not having done something bad, but being incapable of helping children or others in need), and seeing the future as bleak. Another common maladaptive thought involves the belief that one's actions will lead to catastrophe. In part, these beliefs of helplessness may be reinforced by actions of adult children and others who harp on the person's deficits, as reflected in the "learned helplessness" model (Seligman, 1975). As one patient said, "I cook 100 meals and have no problems, and they [the adult children] say nothing; but if I burn the food once, they try to stop me from cooking anymore. I stopped complaining to keep peace."

The question of whether one can learn optimism and change behaviors by insight has underlain all psychotherapies (Seligman, 1998). Cognitive techniques in CBT are tied to exercises in changing behavior or rehearsing. This approach is different from behavioral therapy (conditioned learning) used in work with patients with dementia, which does not require insight, just intermittent positive reinforcement. The cognitive and behavioral components of CBT are summarized in Table 10.2.

Table 10.2. Cognitive and Behavioral Components of CBT

COGNITIVE (teach pattern recognition, reasoning, and responses to problems)	BEHAVIORAL (practice and reinforce solutions through success)
Patient keeps diary of daily activities identifying: • Situation • Automatic thoughts • Emotions (and how intense) • Evaluation—alternative response ("How much do you believe these automatic thoughts and what can you do differently?") Teach early warning signs of problems Patient learns to appreciate and nurture the social support system Patient learns to use organizing tools to reduce distractibility (e.g., written lists)	Ratings of mastery and pleasure (improvement is the reinforcement) Graded tasks (failure-free activities) Role-playing, assertiveness practice, imagery, rehearsal (exposure, cognitive restructuring) Rehearse ideal behaviors

Source: Adapted from Beck & Newman (2005).

CBT groups seem well accepted by older adults, especially if the group is described as a "Depression Class" and not as "Group Therapy."

Use of CBT in COPD, depression following a stroke, panic disorder, insomnia, and GAD has been reported, including treatment manuals that describe what some do, session by session (Munoz & Miranda, 2000). An example of the focus of a 12-session group on depression over several months might be as follows (Munoz & Miranda, 2000).

Structure:

Session 1:	One-hour introduction, examples, and problem list generation
Session 2:	30-minute session the same week as Session 1
Sessions 3–6:	Begin 30-minute sessions 1 week apart for 4 weeks
Sessions 7–11:	Begin 30-minute sessions 2 weeks apart for 5 sessions
Session 12:	Final session

An outline of possible issues to discuss in each session are listed below:

Stages:

Stage 1:	*Provide introduction.*
	Link symptoms to problems in life.
	Emphasize systematic manner.
	Message: Improvement follows action on problems.
Stage 2:	*Construct problem list.*
	Divide larger problems into smaller, more manageable points.
	Define the problem clearly.
Stage 3:	*Set achievable goals connected to the problem.*
	Goals must be objective and quantifiable—"What do you want to do about the problem?"
Stage 4:	*Generate alternative solutions.*
	Brainstorm as many options as possible.
	Note that ideas must come from the patient; this stage is not about teaching skills.
	Withhold judgment during this stage.

Stage 5:   *Choose a preferred solution that best meets the patient's needs* (i.e., best net yield).

Utility assessment—apply a decision tree strategy.

Stage 6:   *Make a step-by-step plan for resolution.*

Have specific homework tasks.

Plan around obstacles.

Stage 7:   *Evaluate progress.*

Point out links between acting on problems, problem resolution, and symptom change.

Antidepressive medications are usually required and although not the focus of the group, are monitored after the group sessions.

Interpersonal Psychotherapy

Interpersonal psychotherapy (ITP) is a method of treating depression that uses several techniques that resemble CBT. It involves weekly sessions over 3–4 months. Initial sessions are generally diagnostic, using active listening; middle sessions address problematic relationship areas, often utilizing role-playing and communication analysis; and final sessions focus on termination formulated as another loss experience from which patients can learn (how they feel, how to use insights to cope differently with the loss this time). The focus is always on interpersonal issues, and the goal is to help patients generate their own interventions.

Therapists who have not been supervised in using the technique often select inappropriate clients, have difficulty clarifying the contract and expectations, deviate from the focus (e.g., allowing long exploration of developmental issues or talking too much about medication), and are too passive in sessions (International Society for Interpersonal Psychotherapy, 2006).

Dialectical Behavior Therapy

Dialectical behavior therapy (DBT) is a form of CBT described initially by Linehan and colleagues (1991) for borderline patients but which has been expanded to other therapeutic contexts, including the treatment of depression in older adults. Riegel (1976) was a forerunner in this areas, describing problems of late life as dialectical dilemmas. Dialecticism is a philosophical abstraction of Georg Hegel (1770–1831), who described the triad of "thesis, antithesis, synthesis" underlying social situations. A thesis (e.g., a person's stated position) would cause the creation of an opposition (antithesis), which would eventually result in a synthesis. In older adults, dialectical dilemmas involve differences between desire and actual situations (e.g., accepting elements of life that cannot be changed), being aware of things of which one disapproves without being judgmental, wanting to concentrate better, tolerating pain, acting opposite to the way one wants to be, and wanting to achieve interpersonal effectiveness (Lynch et al., 2003). Lynch's model involves weekly half-hour individual sessions and 2-hour group sessions that teach distress-tolerance skills and emotion regulation to tolerate suicidal ideation, strong negative emotions, and distressing memories and situations; labeling of emotions; and weekly homework assignments to monitor depressive situations.

Behavioral Therapy for Patients with Cognitive Impairment

Elderly people with mild to more severe cognitive impairment appear more concrete and repetitious or have executive function deficits (judgment problems). The psychotherapeutic procedures that have evolved for work with cognitively impaired individuals generally follow behavioral therapy (reinforcement, extinction) models rather than CBT, because dementia patients generally lack verbal skills or insight (see Chapter 4). Procedural learning seems to remain relatively intact in AD until very late in the course of illness.

CASE EXAMPLE

Mrs. Z is a 74-year-old woman with AD. She wanders and tries to leave day care, shows minimal insight, and can recall none of three words on the MMSE. The patient learned to go to the day room (which was relabeled the living room) by taking repeated walks in which the endpoint was the day room, where she was offered a snack and increased pleasant social time with staff. She stopped wandering within a week. The exit door was disguised by the same color paint as the walls to reduce the patient's notice of it.

Table 10.3 provides a summary of the therapies covered in this section and typically used with older adults.

Table 10.3. Profiles of Therapies Commonly Used with Older Adults

TYPE OF THERAPY	GOALS	WHO MIGHT BENEFIT	SUITABLE FOR COGNITIVELY IMPAIRED?
Psychodynamic psychotherapy (long-term)	Primary goals: increased self-awareness, objective capacity for self-observation Secondary goals: symptom relief (comes with insight), improved relationships Relational based (interpretation of transference)	Psychologically minded individuals who feel conflicted about past	No
CBT (cognitive-behavioral therapy) (3–4 months)	Primary goal: recognize and change automatic thoughts Secondary goal: symptom relief (comes with altered thoughts and newly learned alternative behaviors) Cognitively based (reasoning)	Wide range of cases with the common wish to change behaviors	No
IPT (interpersonal psychotherapy) (3–4 months)	Primary goal: change social functioning that leads to symptoms Secondary goal: improvement of depression Interpersonal focus (transference is not the main focus)	Those whose conflicts center on interpersonal disputes, role transitions, grief or interpersonal deficits	No

Table 10.3. (continued)

TYPE OF THERAPY	GOALS	WHO MIGHT BENEFIT	SUITABLE FOR COGNITIVELY IMPAIRED?
DBT (dialectical behavioral therapy) (2–4 months)	Primary goal: accept synthesis of two opposite thoughts Secondary goal: symptom relief of depression Mixed cognitive and experiential aspects	Those who are disapproving of self and wish to stop unwanted behaviors	No
Reminiscence therapy (2–4 months)	Primary goals: reappraisal of beliefs and life defining events, identify past coping skills Secondary goal: life satisfaction, symptom relief Free association without interpretation	Those with perceived life crisis and dementia patients (lost memories)	Yes

GRIEF AND MOURNING

Although loss and one's own death are normal parts of life, death still comes as a surprise and is not readily accepted by most of us. The older literature on death, dying, and mourning remains the major reference source on patterns of mourning and psychotherapy. The well known Kubler-Ross (1969) model for understanding reactions to the realization of death was observed in cancer patients in the terminal phase of illness. It involves the progression of feelings from denial to anger to depression to bargaining to acceptance. However, it does not reflect how older adults cope with gradual decline or how mourners react to the loss of a loved one.

As with any source of stress, most people cope with death adequately, but many show chronic grief symptoms that devolve into depression. Older widows seem to show a lower rate of major depression than younger widows. Still, 14% of older adults have major depression even 2 years after the loss of a spouse (American

Association for Geriatric Psychiatry, 2005). It is noteworthy that the failure to show marked sadness or distress after a loss, commonly seen as denial, is not a major warning sign of future pathology. Such individuals who do not grieve need not be encouraged to experience grief.

Table 10.4 describes the signs of complicated grief to look for. These are primarily evidence that the patient talks as if the deceased is still alive in their minds.

Table 10.4. Behaviors Seen in Complicated Grief

- Clings to hope that the dead person will return (pining, preoccupations with the dead person, interest in reincarnation, preoccupation with obituaries).
- Tries to see the lost person in someone else.
- Has dreams with representative themes (e.g., frozen in time, dead person is in a struggle for life, sees a dead body without decay).
- Shows primitive defenses (splitting, introjection, identification with deceased).
- Shows externalization (keeps transitional objects—"mummification").

Source: Based on Bowlby (1980).

Table 10.5 describes the premorbid characteristics that predispose one to pathological grief. The major predictors are unexpected death and certain personality predispositions, such as patients with rage, ambivalence, or guilt surrounding the deceased, or unresolved dependency themes (Horowitz et al., 1993).

Table 10.5. Risk Factors for Developing Pathological Grief

SITUATIONAL (UNEXPECTED)
1. Sudden death
2. Delayed mourning
3. Quarrels with relatives and others
4. Attempt to escape the scene
5. Developmental problems ("unsettled" childhood)
6. Suppression (bottled-up feelings)
7. Finding no one helpful

PERSONALITY AND RELATIONSHIP FEATURES
1. Dependent (oral personality); relies on the strong for nurturance
2. Ambivalent relationships
3. Compulsive caregiving disposition
4. Particular marital patterns

Table 10.5. (continued)

- "Cat-and-dog" marriages
- "Babes in the wood" marriages (symbiotic)
5. Avoidance or disavowal of affectional need or ties

Source: Based on Bowlby (1980).

The goals of grief counseling are to increase the reality of the loss, encourage a healthy withdrawal from the deceased, and encourage a reinvestment in other relationships. The methods basically focus on helping the patient deal with affect (both expressed and latent), and overcome impediments to readjustment after the loss (Worden, 1982). Table 10.6 summarizes the typical steps in grief counseling.

Table 10.6. Typical Steps in Grief Counseling

- Encourage patient to talk freely and at length about circumstances leading to the death and experiences after it.
- Later, encourage patient to talk about the person who is lost (first meeting, ups and downs) and perhaps even show photographs, etc.
- Encourage patient to cry and express affect ("It's good that you're letting go").
- Explore and defuse "linking objects" (items that the patient carries all the time as a reminder, usually clothing or jewelry).
- Help direct the stages of mourning to follow this sequence:
  ✓ Idealization first
  ✓ Guilt and anger later
  ✓ Acceptance
- Interpret or point out pathological defenses or patterns (e.g., inhibition, anger, misdirected guilt).
- Ask what it would be like to end grieving. What does he or she see for the future?
- Help the patient say a final goodbye.
- Encourage planning next steps (new relationships, new experiences).

Source: Based on Bowlby (1980) and Worden (1982).

Often patients wrongly think that moving out of grieving means that they will forget the deceased, and that it is a betrayal to the deceased to let go. It is usually helpful to reassure patients that the outcome of grieving is that they won't forget, but when they think about the deceased, it should make them feel good, not bad. Sad thoughts about the person will no longer torment them but will still be accessible.

GROUP THERAPY

Special groups for the elderly usually focus on dealing with depression, developing stress management skills, improving social skills and decreasing isolation, reminiscence (especially for patients with early dementia), and reducing agitation in dementia (see Chapter 4). Group approaches for the cognitively intact may be divided into verbal-centered groups, creativity- and activity-centered groups (e.g., dance-movement, drama, art, poetry, project groups), and service or self-help groups (Leszcz, 2004). The last two categories are generally considered social or educational groups and would not be covered by Medicare.

Group therapy is not advised for patients who are in acute crisis, are paranoid or violent, or have severe communication problems (e.g., deaf, overly sedated). Indications for group therapy rather than individual therapy are social isolation, interpersonal alienation, maladaptive interpersonal skills, diminished self-worth, depressive disengagement, and withdrawal. Group therapy may be more acceptable and less anxiety provoking than individual therapy for such individuals because dependence may be diminished and affect is diffused among others who share their concerns and the limelight. However, these are also the same factors that older adults typically give when resisting group participation: "I'm a loner," "I hate being with people." Preparation and pretraining of patients prior to entry into group therapy may be necessary, although this area has not been researched in older adults. This may involve providing information and explaining the rationale of group therapy, or even a brief role-playing of what interactions in a group might be like. In any case, the therapist carries a greater responsibility to initiate and activate the group than is typical of a group composed of younger patients (Leszcz, 2004).

Group settings such as day hospitals and intensive outpatient programs (IOPs) are increasingly utilized by older adults. The groups seem most effective when they are composed only of elderly people—that is, not age-mixed—because pacing, core themes and concerns, and establishing group cohesion is more likely to be shared with peers. Group therapy is not the same as social groups, and the specific therapeutic function and approach to achieve the group goals must be carefully considered, just as with younger patients.

SUMMARY

In doing therapy with older adults, special attention must be paid to countertransference (e.g., ageism) in the therapist and to regressive behaviors by the patient (e.g., splitting) and the need for limit setting—patients must come to sessions, not call between sessions, and not create dissension among caregivers, such as family members. Pacing, degree of insight, communication style, and themes make psychotherapy different for older adults, but the same major approaches are used: psychodynamic psychotherapy, CBT, ITP, reminiscence therapy, and group psychotherapy. Special techniques, especially behavior therapy with reinforcement contingencies, are applied to patients who have dementia with behavior problems.

11

PSYCHIATRY IN THE NURSING HOME AND INPATIENT CARE

Locations of practice have different patient case mixes and problems, different organization and staffing, and different roles for the psychiatrist. Many psychiatrists view their role in these settings as solely diagnosis and medication management of major psychiatric disorders; they do not address psychotherapy needs, the treatment milieu, interpersonal conflicts, staff or family interventions or training. Needless to say, treatment outcomes are worse if the basic stressors do not change, and no active psychosocial intervention is offered. Many of the behavioral disturbances in patients with dementia, for example, are not responsive to medications, and rehospitalization occurs quickly if the only treatment offered is calming of acute agitation by medications during a hospital stay.

NURSING HOME AND LONG-TERM CARE WORK WITH OLDER ADULTS

Although the percentage of persons over 65 who reside in nursing homes has been remarkably constant over the years, at about 5%, the average age of nursing home residents has continued to rise with the increased longevity of the general population. The name "retirement home" has been supplanted by the term "assisted living," but nursing homes for the more medically impaired and patients with dementia remain hospital-like facilities. Although medical outcomes for many health issues, such as bedsores, gross patient abuse or neglect, and reduction in antipsychotic medication use, have improved since nursing home reform provisions were passed in 1987 (the Omnibus Budget Reconciliation Act [OBRA]), little seems to have changed in psychosocial care within nursing homes. They are still far from "homelike settings" (Seaton, 2002).

The need for psychiatric services within nursing home settings has never been greater. Although estimates are available from Minimum Data Set (MDS), data may underrepresent the problem, because MDS ratings of psychiatric symptoms are often performed by an MDS nurse who completes the forms with minimal direct interaction with the patients. An earlier study applying a semistructured Diagnostic Interview Schedule (DIS) to all residents in two Minnesota nursing homes showed an 84% prevalence of Axis I DSM-III psychiatric diagnoses (Teeter et al., 1976). Yet, in a typical nursing home, consultation requests seem to be limited to severe behavioral disturbances. More mild impairment, including moderate depression, is often untreated (Fenton, et al., 2004).

Federal regulations for nursing home reform, which were enacted by Congress in response to a scathing Institute of Medicine (1986) report on the quality of nursing home care, contained three main psychiatric provisions:

1. *Elimination of unnecessary use of restraints.* Initially, chemical restraints included any psychotropic medication, but this was quickly changed to accept psychotropics for therapeutic indications (see Adams's summary of OBRA regulations, 1999). Restraints do not significantly decrease behavioral disturbance and potentially increase agitation, falls, injuries, skin breakdowns, and functional decline (Werner et al., 1989).

2. *PASARR (pre-admission screening and annual review of residents).* Patients entering a nursing facility that accepts Medicaid require certification that the patient is not being admitted for a primary psychiatric diagnosis. Psychiatric patients are to be treated in an institution for mental disease. Each state's review process is different (i.e., forms and rating groups differ). Initially the review was to be repeated annually, but re-review is now needed only after leaving the facility, such as for a psychiatric hospitalization.

3. *The MDS has two pages of psychiatric information that need to be filled out in detail initially,* with quarterly updates. Potentially unnecessary psychiatric medications include antipsychotic medication without psychosis, or regular anxiolytic or hypnotic medication (more than 2x/week).

Nursing Home Model

Ideally, psychiatry should be a part of the care team, such as in a consultation–liaison model applied within the nursing home (Sakauye, 1992). The teaching nursing home model involves residents and fellows liaisoning with nursing home staff in structured weekly "rounds" in a nursing home. In a 103-bed, not-for-profit, religious nursing home in an urban area, the program clearly led to decreased psychiatric hospitalization rates, decreased psychotropic polypharmacy, decreased staff complaints, and improved patient response. The same positive outcome is seen in larger nursing homes and may involve nurse practitioners or social workers.

A recommended schedule in this nursing home model involves the following:

- Initial nursing rounds with the coordinator who handles the schedule.
- Patient sessions in the patient's room or an office that offers privacy (billable services—patients referred by their physicians).
- Informal patient contacts—patients have a question or introduce MDs to new patients (not billed).
- Programs for patients (e.g., discussant at an afternoon tea).
- Staff-directed consultations (questions about patients, treatment planning, explaining meds).
- Staff training and case-based discussions. (In facilities with stable staff we met with four different staff groupings for 30 minutes; this allowed all of the staff to participate in a monthly meeting on psychosocial issues without disturbing patient care; Sakauye, 1992.)
- Exit interview with the coordinator (may involve other interested staff)—review recommendations, follow up on sessions,

and ensure that recommendations will be entered into patients' care plans.

In order to reduce the stigma of "talking to a shrink," make initial introductions to each new patient as one of the facility doctors and offer to help during this difficult transition phase. This prior introduction reduces resistance later if the patient is referred. In addition, being a guest at the resident's council or some social function during rounds is helpful in reducing stigma.

Typical Case Mix

A 1-year analysis of the case mix of consultations in this teaching nursing home model that our university undertook was as follows:

- About 50% of patients in the facility were referred.
- 47% of patients were seen no more than twice (consultation only).
- Only 6% of patients were seen once a month or more.
- No psychiatric hospitalizations were required.

Table 11.1 presents the percent of referrals in our university program by diagnosis.

Table 11.1. Percent of Referrals by Diagnosis

DIAGNOSIS	% OF REFERRALS
Dementia (290.xx, 291.2, 294.xx)	41.6%
Mood Disorders (296.xx, 311.0)	34.9%
Anxiety Disorders (300.xx)	8.9%
Psychotic Disorders (295.xx, 297.x, 298.x)	6.3%
Adjustment Disorder (309.xx)	5.4%
Other (e.g., impulse control, personality disorders, sleep disorders, noncompliance)	1.5%
Total	100%

The goals for the program were as follows:

- Identify and treat causes of delirium.
- Verify dementia diagnoses (review records and repeat mental status evaluations); order tests as appropriate.
- Evaluate medications for possible medication interactions and adverse effects.
- Optimize psychotropic medication (rules to minimize polypharmacy and excess dosing).
- Define a psychosocial treatment plan, especially for dementia.
- Provide short-term counseling or refer for long-term psychotherapy, when needed.
- Supervise and educate staff around psychosocial issues and monitoring guidelines for psychotropic medications.
- Convey suggestions about milieu improvement (home-like rather than hospital-like setting, reorienting cues, staff behavior, communicating with sensory-impaired or dementia patients).

Dementia Units

Special care units such as Alzheimer's units have been established in about 22% of U.S. nursing homes (Streim & Katz, 2004). These are generally locked units for ambulatory, behaviorally disturbed Alzheimer's patients. In order to reduce violence or need for restraints, units are safety proofed, have activity programs and exercise, reorientation cues, higher staff ratios, and "wandering" space. Usually, psychiatric assistance is needed in establishing a therapeutic milieu, advising on behavioral management, and monitoring cognitive and psychotropic medications. The psychiatric approach to diagnosis or treatment does not change, but psychiatric involvement does require taking a leadership role in defining optimal psychosocial care and educating nonpsychiatric staff.

Reimbursement Issues

In this type of consultation–liaison program about 33% of time is spent providing nonbillable services (education, "curbside consults"). Billable services are covered at 50% of approved rates under traditional Medicare, which still pays 80% of 62.5% of the approved rate. Current approved rates for each region are published on the CMS website (Centers for Medicare and Medicaid Services; www.cms.hhs.gov/FeeScheduleGenInfo). The co-insurance portion is often not affordable to many nursing home residents. Often there is no co-insurance and Medicaid only pays up to its limit, not the full co-payment. Managed Medicare companies usually pay below Medicare approved rates, although they generally pay 80%, not 50%.

Because of the high amount of nonreimbursed time, it is prudent to establish a contract for the estimated nonreimbursable hours (possibly for 33% of the time) as a consultant or psychiatric medical director. When such reimbursement is not available, we have advocated donating limited time as community service to "adopt a home." There is partial reimbursement and this is a necessary effort. For teaching programs, the time may be covered indirectly through the Graduate Medical Education (GME) mechanism that pays part of attending salaries plus resident stipends. An occasional home may decide to add a surcharge to all patients' monthly bills to cover the contract. A few choose to cover consultant fees in a contract and not allow billing. Some programs also use psychiatric nurse practitioners with psychiatrist backup because there is reimbursement for this, and the expense is less.

Some Medicare carriers do not allow electronic billing for Medicare services provided by consultants in nursing homes because they require a copy of the signed order and consult note to be appended for payment (100% review). Although these measures delay payment and increase the cost of billing, this is a necessary service for patients and hopefully can be provided. Some Medicare changes are a result of Operation Restore Trust. This was a two-year anti-fraud and abuse project initiated in May, 1995 in California, Florida, Illinois, New York, and Texas, though additional states came on board later. The project imposed harsher documentation standards on issues surrounding home health, nursing homes, hospice, and medical equipment and supplies. It also required specific signed orders accompanied by a copy of the psychiatry note in order for payment to be issued.

INPATIENT HOSPITAL CARE, PARTIAL HOSPITALIZATION, INTENSIVE OUTPATIENT PROGRAM

Psychiatric Care requires a continuum of care from outpatient care, which has been the main focus of earlier chapters, to nursing home care. This section deals with how to determine the optimal level of care in between these modalities.

One way of determining the level of care a patient needs is the current Global Assessment of Function (GAF), or Axis V in the DSM IV-TR. Inpatient hospitalization is usually needed when the GAF is 35 or less. Functioning at this level is impaired in reality testing or communication (e.g., speech is at times illogical, obscure, or irrelevant), or major impairment exists in several areas such as family relationships, judgment, thinking, or mood (e.g., inability to complete tasks) (American Psychiatric Association, 2000). A GAF score between 35 and 45 may require an intermediate program like a partial hospitalization (day hospital), an intensive outpatient program (IOP), or excellent social support. Inpatient admission for GAF scores above 35 may still be needed if a suicide risk is present, even in the presence of reasonable social supports and intermediate resources. Table 11.2 summarizes the criteria used for admission to a geriatric psychiatry inpatient unit.

Table 11.2. Geriatric Psychiatry Inpatient Criteria

CORE PSYCHIATRIC SYMPTOMS (one must be present)	SECONDARY NEED FOR INPATIENT TREATMENT (one must be present in addition to a core symptom)	RELATIVE CONTRAINDICATIONS TO ADMISSION
Severe affective disorder	Severity: Homicidal Suicidal Gravely disabled	Bedbound (no need for a locked unit)
Severe psychotic disorder		Unstable medical condition (where daily rounds by internal medicine and daily changes in medication or IV orders are needed)
Severe behavioral disorder in dementia or delirium requiring a locked unit for management (redirection, activity programs, ADIs, and reorientation retraining)	Inadequate outpatient treatment (failure of or inability to get to outpatient services)	
	Refusal of help due to psychiatric condition (thought disorder)	
Severe behavioral disorder requiring restraints (attempt to decrease restraint use by psychiatric medication management and a less medical supportive milieu)	Need to establish or shore up an outpatient support network to allow outpatient treatment to proceed (active social work involvement)	

Note. ADIs = activities of daily living.

The clinical purpose of a geriatric psychiatry inpatient unit separate from the general adult unit is mainly patient safety. In many acute care facilities, the elderly must be protected from more violent younger patients. A second, nearly equally important reason is to provide age-appropriate programming. Geriatric units deal with different themes, have more family involvement, pace programs and exercise differently, have more medical coverage, and allow for dementia care.

On most geriatric units there is still a wide range of diagnoses and functional abilities. Cognitively intact depressed elderly will need different programs than regressed, agitated, or demented patients. To accommodate this, geriatric units should be able to provide at least two tracks, one for higher functioning elderly and another for lower functioning elderly patients. Table 11.3 provides a sample program on a geriatric psychiatric unit.

Table 11.3. Sample Program on a Geriatric Psychiatry Unit

	HIGHER FUNCTIONING (typical geropsychiatric patient)	LOWER FUNCTIONING (dementia, severely regressed)
A.M.	Medical tests and evaluations Individual psychiatry sessions Group psychotherapy	Physical care needs Medical tests and evaluations Functional testing (OT) Individual psychiatry sessions
P.M.	Group therapies—two or three sessions per day Nursing Psychology Social Work Recreation: Movies Discussion groups Television (with discussion) Reading Internet, TV or other isolative activities are usually avoided.	Continuous activity programming with shorter groups Emphasis on "interaction" and modeling ADIs retraining Medication management Family work (social work) Possible placement preparation

Note. ECT may be required for either group. OT = occupational therapy; ADIs = activities of daily living.

For patients with dementia, it is important to compress the diagnostic workup into as short a period as possible. Each discipline must be clear about its role in the diagnostic process so that information can be shared and a definitive treatment plan made quickly. If a patient has been referred from a nursing home and is on Medicaid, the home does not get paid to hold the bed beyond 5 working days. Nursing homes become reluctant to refer if prolonged hospital stays routinely exceed their reimbursed period. The primary responsibility for the care plan is still in the hands of the psychiatrist, but social work needs to work intensively with the family and/or referring nursing home; OT should assess functional capacity and the patient's capacity for maximum function; and geriatric medicine should review and stabilize medical issues and medication regimens. The key issues are to (1) confirm diagnosis, (2) do functional staging, and (3) expand support network. Table 4.10 summarizes a hospital workup procedure for patients with dementia and behavioral disturbance.

With the growing need for shorter lengths of stay, "step-down programs" become increasingly important. Patients are discharged early with follow-up in a day hospital or Intensive Outpatient Program (IOP) as soon as possible. Day hospitals are scheduled like the day shift of a hospital, and supervision at home is provided at night and weekends for patients without dementia. Generally, patients with dementia must have either supportive care through adult day-care or home health assistance if there is family to supervise, because Medicare usually will not approve psychotherapy programs for patients with dementia. IOPs usually work with patients two or three times per week, instead of daily, for shorter lengths of time as an alternative to day hospitals.

Reimbursement Issues

Medicare covers 100% of the hospital daily rate and medications under Medicare Part A. Day hospital and IOP daily rates are also covered under Part A, but medications are not. Physician fees, under Medicare Part B, are covered at 80% of approved rates for inpatient care but only 50% for outpatient care. Outpatient payments are defined as 80% of 62.5% of approved charges. Medication benefits vary under Medicare Part D (drug coverage). Benefits differ for managed Medicare companies because they have a waiver to apply their own rules as long as overall range of services is the same as traditional Medicare (Group for the Advancement of Psychiatry, 2005). These companies have their own review or prior authorization criteria, unlike Medicare, which has a retrospective review triggered by internal criteria.

Patients seem most comfortable when the treating physician is in charge of their care in all locations, and they do not have a different doctor in charge whenever they change from outpatient to inpatient, to IOP, to nursing home. Taking measures to ensure that records are shared is the only way to minimize disruption in care plans if the ideal of having one physician in charge in all settings cannot be achieved.

SUMMARY

Medicare has different reimbursement criteria for psychiatry in nursing homes and inpatient care. Many intermediaries still believe that dementia patients do not require psychiatric intervention. If not approved, care should be appealed and careful attention to coding and documentation must be maintained. Inpatient and outpatient settings vary widely from intensive care to step-down units to long-term care in the home or in a residential setting. Inpatient hospital care is usually restricted to patients with a GAF score of 35 or less. To best organize care in each setting, the psychiatrist must lead a multidisciplinary team involved in patient care and serve as a liaison with other physicians. This part is time-consuming and usually requires a separate administrative contract as a consultant or medical director.

APPENDIX 1

CLINICAL ASSESSMENT FORMS

PSYCHIATRY CONSULTATION ORDER FORM

This is to certify that _____ was evaluated by me and requires psychiatric care for the following reason/reasons (check all that apply):

__ Depression, nonresponsive to an antidepressant trial

— Severe depression, evaluate for hospitalization

— Severe agitation in dementia
  __ Will require hospitalization if not improved soon
  __ Will require assistance in behavior plan to reduce restraints
  __ Will require psychotropic medication

__ Presence of delusions or hallucinations

— Psychiatric medication review (continue, discontinue, reduce number, evaluate dosage)

— Severe anxiety

__ Tranquilizer dependence

__ Maintenance for a chronic medically ill patient (schizophrenia, bipolar disorder, etc.)

__ Other (specify): _____

I would like:

__Consultation and recommendations only

— Ongoing psychiatric treatment (treatment plan to be reviewed by me)

_____   _____
Attending signature   Date

PREVISIT QUESTIONNAIRES

History Review of Cognitive Changes: Dementia Assessment Profile

Patient Name:

1. When did you first notice confusion or memory problems?

2. What were the first symptoms?

3. Did symptoms get worse gradually, or were there sharp turns? Describe briefly:

4. When did you first seek medical help for the problem?

5. Is there a family history of dementia or senility? Who (what relationship)?

6. Have you ever been a heavy drinker? Had head trauma causing a concussion? Had a seizure disorder?

7. Have you ever had a CT scan or MRI of the head? When? Where?

8. Have you ever had an EEG? When? Where?

9. What diagnosis have you been given for the cognitive problem? By whom? What specialty?

10. Do you have a history of depression or other psychiatric problem? Describe:

11. When did the behavior problems begin? What approaches have helped reduce the problems?

12. What medications are you aware of that have been tried for the behavior problems?

NEUROLOGICAL EXAMINATION SUMMARY
GERIATRIC PSYCHIATRY

CRANIAL NERVES		INTACT	ABNORMAL (Describe)
Olfactory I	Smells freshly burned match, fresh coffee, or alcohol swab		
Optic II	Distinguishes object (each eye separately) Distinguishes movements in peripheral field		
Oculomotor III Trochlear IV Abducens VI	Gazes symmetrically up, down, sideways		
Trigeminal V	Distinguishes one- from two-point touch symmetrically on forehead, cheeks, and chin; chews symmetrically		
Facial VII	Upper: frowns symmetrically Lower: smiles symmetrically		
Auditory VIII	Hears finger rubbing or snapping equally in both ears		
Glossopharyngeal IX	Has symmetrical gag reflex or uvula midline		
Vagus X	Can make guttural sounds		
Accessory XI	Shrugs shoulders symmetrically Can resist turning of head symmetrically		
Hyoglossal XII	Can stick tongue out straight; no atrophy of tongue		

Gross Neurological Exam

Sensory/Motor Functions:

Coordination:

Deep Tendon Reflexes:

Pathological Reflexes:

Physician's Signature: _____

Date: _____ Time: _____

FUNCTIONAL EVALUATION IN DEMENTIA

Check all that apply:

ADAPTIVE SKILLS

_____ Needs help handling money
_____ Needs help bathing
_____ Dresses inappropriately
_____ Needs help dressing
_____ Gets confused in new places
_____ Misses meals/doesn't eat
_____ Needs help walking
_____ Has bathroom accidents

ORIENTATION

_____ Gets lost in the neighborhood
_____ Difficulty discussing current issues
_____ Gets confused easily when talking with others
_____ Needs help telling time
_____ Needs help remembering dates such as birthdays/holidays

MEMORY

_____ Trouble remembering things
_____ Needs help recalling past life events
_____ Forgets people's names
_____ Forgets to keep appointments
_____ Loses things

SOCIAL FUNCTIONING

_____ Fails to maintain usual contact with family
_____ Needs help conversing
_____ Wanders off topic
_____ Fails to form good sentences
_____ Doesn't talk as much

HALLUCINATIONS/ DELUSIONS

_____ Hears things/voices not there
_____ Sees things/people not there
_____ Tries to strike others
_____ Has paranoid delusions; fears for own safety
_____ Feels superior to others
_____ Believes has great power

AGGRESSION

_____ Becomes aggressive easily
_____ Shouts at others
_____ Throws/breaks objects
_____ Tries to injure self

OCCUPATIONAL FUNCTIONING

_____ Needs help with household chores
_____ Needs help with hobbies
_____ Needs help with phone/dials wrong numbers
_____ Makes mistakes when doing hobbies
_____ Uses tools/appliances wrong
_____ Needs help preparing meals
_____ Needs help using utensils
_____ Rearranges objects needlessly/puts keys in freezer

Source: Adapted from a variety of caregiver surveys.

HEALTH QUESTIONNAIRE

CONDITION (If Yes, write in diagnosis if known)	Yes	No	First noticed when?	Does this limit you in any way?	List the MD you see for this
Eyes					
Ears (especially hearing)					
Nose and Throat					
Endocrine (e.g., thyroid, diabetes)					
Lungs					
Heart					
Gastrointestinal (GI) (e.g., ulcers, gallbladder problems)					
Genitourinary Tract (GU) (e.g., kidneys, uterine problems, prostate problems)					
Stroke					
Seizures					
Other Neurological Problems (e.g., Parkinson's)					
Arthritis					
Osteoporosis					
Cancer (type)					
Anemia/Abnormal Blood					
Allergies					
Substance Use					

Source: Adapted from Duke University Center for the Study of Aging and Human Development (2006).

Comments:

_____

_____

_____

_____

_____

_____

_____

_____

_____

_____

_____

_____

_____

_____

Hospitalizations and Surgeries
(including childhood)

CONDITION	WHEN?	CITY, STATE, & HOSPITAL

Current Doctors

Primary Physician:

Name: _____

Specialty: _____

Address: _____

_____

City: _____ State: _____ Zip Code: _____

Office Phone: _____ Office Fax: _____

Specialists:

Name: _____

Specialty: _____

Address: _____

_____

City: _____ State: _____ Zip Code: _____

Office Phone: _____ Office Fax: _____

Name: _____

Specialty: _____

Address: _____

_____

City: _____ State: _____ Zip Code: _____

Office Phone: _____ Office Fax: _____

Name: _____

Specialty: _____

Address: _____

_____

City: _____ State: _____ Zip Code: _____

Office Phone: _____ Office Fax: _____

Name: _____

Specialty: _____

Address: _____

_____

City: _____ State: _____ Zip Code: _____

Office Phone: _____ Office Fax: _____

Current Medication List

MEDICATION	DOSE	WHEN TAKEN?	SIDE EFFECTS?

Comments:

Previous Psychiatric Medications

*Please list all past psychiatric medications used in order,
from the earliest to the most recent:*

MEDICATION	APPROX. DATES USED	MAX DAILY DOSE	PRESCRIBING DOCTOR

Examples of common psychiatric medicines
(to jog your memory)

SSRIs

Fluoxetine (Prozac, Serafem)
Citalopram (Celexa)
Escitalopram (Lexapro)
Paroxetine (Prozac, Pexeva)
Sertraline (Zoloft)
Fluvoxemine (Luvox)
Symbyax (combination med.)

Other Antidepressants

Imipramine (Tofranil)
Amitriptyline (Elavil, Endep)
Desipramine (Norpramin)
Nortriptyline (Pamelor, Aventy)
Doxepin (Sinequan, Adepin)
Trimipramine (Surmontil)
Protriptyline (Vivactil)
Clomipramine (Anafranil)
Limbitrol (combination med.)
Triavil (combination med.)
Methylphenidate (Ritalin)
Amoxepine (Ascendin)

Mirtazapine (Remeron)
Trazadone (Desyrel)
Bupropion (Wellbutrin)
Maprotaline (Ludiomil)
Venlafaxine (Effexor)
Nefazadone (Serzone)
Duloxetine (Cymbalta)

MAOIs

Tranylcypromine (Parnate)
Phenelzine (Nardil)
Isocarboxazid (Marplan)

Atypical Antipsychotics

Quetiapine (Seroquel)
Risperidone (Risperdal)
Olanzapine (Zyprexa, Zydis)
Ziprasidone (Geodon)
Clozapine (Clozaril)
Aripiprazole (Abilify)

Typical Antipsychotics

Haloperidol (Haldol)
Fluphenazine (Prolinxin)
Trifluoperazine (Stelazine)
Perphenazine (Trilafon)
Thioridazine (Mellaril)
Chlorpromazine (Thorazine)
Thiothixene (Navane)

Pimizide (Orap)
Mesoridazine (Serentil)
Molindone (Moban)
Loxapine (Loxitane)
Triavil (combination med.)

Anxiety & Sleeping Meds

Alprazolam (Xanax)
Lorazepam (Ativan)
Oxazepam (Serax)
Buspirone (BuSpar)
Meprobamate
Clorazepate (Tranxene)
Diazepam (Valium)
Chlordiazepoxide (Librium)
Clonazepam (Klonopin)
Limbitrol (combination med.)

Sleeping Meds

Zaleplon (Sonata)
Zolpidem (Ambien)
Eszopiclone (Lunesta)
Ramelteon (Rozerem)
Triazolam (Halcion)
Estazolam (Prodomm)
Flurazepam (Dalmane)
Temazepam (Restoril)
Hydroxyzine (Atarax, Vistaril)

Table A.1. Body Mass Index (BMI) Table

	NORMAL							OVERWEIGHT							OBESE				
BMI	19	20	21	22	23	24	25	26	27	28	29	30	31	32	33	34	35	36
Height (inches)				Body Weight (pounds)														
58	91	96	100	105	110	115	119	124	129	134	138	143	148	153	158	162	167	
59	94	99	104	109	114	119	124	128	133	138	143	148	153	158	163	168	173	
60	97	102	107	112	118	123	128	133	138	143	148	153	158	163	168	174	179	
61	100	106	111	116	122	127	132	137	143	148	153	158	164	169	174	180	185	
62	104	109	115	120	126	131	136	142	147	153	158	164	169	175	180	186	191	
63	107	113	118	124	130	135	141	146	152	158	163	169	175	180	186	191	197	
64	110	116	122	128	134	140	145	151	157	163	169	174	180	186	192	197	204	
65	114	120	126	132	138	144	150	156	162	168	174	180	186	192	198	204	210	
66	118	124	130	136	142	148	155	161	167	173	179	186	192	198	204	210	216	
67	121	127	134	140	146	153	159	166	172	178	185	191	198	204	211	217	223	
68	125	131	138	144	151	158	164	171	177	184	190	197	203	210	216	223	230	
69	128	135	142	149	155	162	169	176	182	189	196	203	209	216	223	230	236	
70	132	139	146	153	160	167	174	181	188	195	202	209	216	222	229	236	243	
71	136	143	150	157	165	172	179	186	193	200	208	215	222	229	236	243	250	
72	140	147	154	162	169	177	184	191	199	206	213	221	228	235	242	250	258	
73	144	151	159	166	174	182	189	197	204	212	219	227	235	242	250	257	265	
74	148	155	163	171	179	186	194	202	210	218	225	233	241	249	256	264	272	
75	152	160	168	176	184	192	200	208	216	224	232	240	248	256	264	272	279	
76	156	164	172	180	189	197	205	213	221	230	238	246	254	263	271	279	287	

Source: National Heart, Lung, and Blood Institute (2007). Adapted from Clinical Guideline on the Identification, Evaluation, and Treatment of Overweight and Obese Adults: The Evidence Report.

EXTREME OBESITY

	37	38	39	40	41	42	43	44	45	46	47	48	49	50	51	52	53	54
172	177	181	186	191	196	201	205	210	215	220	224	229	234	239	244	248	253	258
178	183	188	193	198	203	208	212	217	222	227	232	237	242	247	252	257	262	267
184	189	194	199	204	209	215	220	225	230	235	240	245	250	255	261	266	271	276
190	195	201	206	211	217	222	227	232	238	243	248	254	259	264	269	275	280	285
196	202	207	213	218	224	229	235	240	246	251	256	262	267	273	278	284	289	295
203	208	214	220	225	231	237	242	248	254	259	265	270	278	282	287	293	299	304
209	215	221	227	232	238	244	250	256	262	267	273	279	285	291	296	302	308	314
216	222	228	234	240	246	252	258	264	270	276	282	288	294	300	306	312	318	324
223	229	235	241	247	253	260	266	272	278	284	291	297	303	309	315	322	328	334
230	236	242	249	255	261	268	274	280	287	293	299	306	312	319	325	331	338	344
236	243	249	256	262	269	276	282	289	295	302	308	315	322	328	335	341	348	354
243	250	257	263	270	277	284	291	297	304	311	318	324	331	338	345	351	358	365
250	257	264	271	278	285	292	299	306	313	320	327	334	341	348	355	362	369	376
257	265	272	279	286	293	301	308	315	322	329	338	343	351	358	365	372	379	386
265	272	279	287	294	302	309	316	324	331	338	346	353	361	368	375	383	390	397
272	280	288	295	302	310	318	325	333	340	348	355	363	371	378	386	393	401	408
280	287	295	303	311	319	326	334	342	350	358	365	373	381	389	396	404	412	420
287	295	303	311	319	327	335	343	351	359	367	375	383	391	399	407	415	423	431
295	304	312	320	328	336	344	353	361	369	377	385	394	402	410	418	426	435	443

APPENDIX 2

RECOMMENDED READING

General Textbooks on Aging

Sadavoy J, Jarvik LF, Grossberg GT, Meyers BS (Eds.): *Comprehensive Textbook of Geriatric Psychiatry* (3rd ed.). New York, Norton, 2004.

Cheong JA (Ed.): *Geriatric Psychiatry Self-Assessment Program (Question Book and Critique Book)*. Bethesda, MD, American Association for Geriatric Psychiatry, 2004.

Bengston VL, WK Schaie (Eds.): *Handbook of Theories of Aging*. New York, Springer, 1999.

Birren J & Schaie KW (Eds.): *Handbook of the Psychology of Aging* (5th ed). San Diego, Academic Press, 2001.

Binstock RH & George LK (Eds.): *Handbook of Aging and the Social Sciences* (5th ed.). San Diego, Academic Press, 2001.

Masoro EJ & Austad S (Eds.): *Handbook of the Biology of Aging* (5th ed). San Diego, Academic Press, 2001.

General Psychiatry Text

Sadock J & Sadock VA (Eds.): *Comprehensive Textbook of Psychiatry* (8th ed.). Baltimore, Lippincott, Williams & Wilkins, 2004.

Diagnostic Criteria

American Psychiatric Association: *Diagnostic and Statistical Manual of Mental Disorders*, Text Revision (4th ed.). Washington, DC, American Psychiatric Association, 2000. (Especially useful items are Appendix A, which provides decision trees for differential diagnosis; Appendix B, which lists proposed new diagnostic categories; and Appendix I, which has an outline for cultural formulation and glossary of culture-bound syndromes.)

Psychopharmacology Textbooks

Hardman JG, Limbird LE, Gillman AG: *Goodman & Gilman's The Phamacological Basis of Therapeutics* (10th ed.). New York, McGraw-Hill, 2001.

Davis KL, Charney D, Coyle JT, Nemeroff C (Eds.): *Neuropsychopharmacology: The Fifth Generation of Progress*. Philadelphia, Lippincott, Williams & Wilkins, 2002.

Stahl SM: *Essential Psychopharmacology: Neuroscientific Basis and Practical Applications* (2nd ed.) New York, Cambridge University Press, 2000.

Psychiatric Services

International Psychogeriatric Association: *Service Delivery Bibliography*. Available at *www.ipa-online.org/pdfs/sdb2005.pdf.* Regularly updated by the Service Delivery Task Force. Initially contained only articles written in English, but is now expanding to include articles written in a variety of languages. Topics covered include architecture, care, economics, legal issues, medication, squalor, structure, and historical development of services. The bibliography covers the last 10 years.

Evidence-Based Practice Guidelines

American Psychiatric Association: *Practice Guidelines*. Available at *www.psych.org/psych_pract/treatg/pg/prac_guide.cfm.*
Texas Department of State Health Services: Texas Treatment Algorithm Project (TMAP). Available at *www.dshs.state.tx.us/mhprograms/disclaimer.shtm.*
Cochrane Collaboration Reviews. Available at *www.cochrane.org/reviews/.* Provides reviews of evidence-based treatments on a variety of topics.

Medicine Textbook

Kasper DL, Braunwald E, Fauci A, Hauser, S, Longo D (Eds.): *Harrison's Principles of Internal Medicine* (16th ed.). New York, McGraw-Hill, 2005.

Genetic Biomarkers

Kendler KS: "A Gene for . . .": The Nature of Gene Action in Psychiatric Disorders. *American Journal of Psychiatry* 162:1243–1252, 2005.
OMIM, Online Mendelian Inheritance in Man. Available at *www.ncbi.nlm.nih.gov/.* Database of human genes and genetic disorders, including subtyping for Alzheimer's disease and many neurological disorders.

Primary Geriatric Psychiatry Journals

American Journal of Geriatric Psychiatry (AJGP)
Journal of the American Geriatrics Society (JAGS)
The Gerontologist (Gerontological Society of America)
The Journals of Gerontology (Gerontological Society of America)
International Psychogeriatrics (International Psychogeriatric Association)
Aging and Mental Health

Recommended Texts for Billing

Schmidt CW Jr., Yowell RK, Jaffe E: *CPT Handbook for Psychiatrists* (3rd ed.). Washington, DC, American Psychiatric Publishing, 2004.
Center for Medicare and Medicaid Services (CMS). Available at *www.cms.hhs.gov/.*

REFERENCES

Adams SR. Unnecessary drugs in the elderly, including the psychotropic utilization protocol: Establishing compliance with the OBRA regulations concerning unnecessary drugs. Dayton, OH: Med-Pass, 1999.

Alexander F, French RM, & Pollock GH. *Psychosomatic specificity, Vol I: Experimental study and results.* Chicago: University of Chicago Press, 1968.

Alexopoulos GS. Vascular disease, depression, and dementia. *American Geriatrics Society* 41:1178–80, 2003.

Alexopoulos GS, Abrams RC, Young RC, & Shamoian CA. Cornell Scale for Depression in Dementia. *Biological Psychiatry* 23(3):271–84, 1988.

Alexopoulos GS, Jeste DV, Chung H, Carpenter D, Ross R, & Docherty JP. Treatment of dementia and its behavioral disturbances: The expert consensus guideline series. *Postgraduate Medicine* (Special Report), January 2005.

Alexopoulos, GS, Meyers BS, Young RC, Campbell D, Silbersweig D, & Charlson M. "Vascular depression" hypothesis. *Arch Gen Psychiatry* 54:915–22, 1997.

Alexopoulos GS, Streim J, Carpenter D, & Docherty JP. Expert consensus panel for using antipsychotic drugs in older patients. *J Clin Psychiatry* 65(Suppl 2):5–99, 2004.

Allen LA, Woolfolk RL, Escobar JI, Gara MA, & Hamer RM. Cognitive–behavioral therapy for somatization disorder: A controlled randomized controlled trial. *Arch Int Medicine* 166:1512–8, 2006.

Alzheimer's Disease Resource Agency of Alaska. Catastrophic reactions. Retrieved February 23, 2006, from *www.alzalaska.org/PDF%20Files/Catostrophic%20reactions%2005.pdf.*

American Academy of Sleep Medicine. *ICSD-international classification of sleep disorders, rev.: Diagnostic and coding manual.* Westchester, IL: American Academy of Sleep Medicine, 2001.

American Association for Geriatric Psychiatry (AAGP). Comment on the U.S. Food and Drug Administration's (FDA) advisory on off-label use of atypical antipsychotics in the elderly. Retrieved April 1, 2005, from *www.aagponline.org/proflantipsychstat_0705.asp.*

American Association for Geriatric Psychiatry. *Late-life depression, progress and hope: Lessons learned from geriatric psychiatry.* Bethesda, MD: American Association for Geriatric Psychiatry, 2004.

American Diabetes Association, American Psychiatric Association, American

Association of Clinical Endocrinologists, North American Association for the Study of Obesity. Consensus development conferences on antipsychotic drugs and obesity and diabetes. *Diabetes Care* 27:596–601, 2004.

American Dietary Association, American Psychiatric Association, American Association of Clinical Endocrinologists, North American Association for the Study of Obesity: Consensus development conference on antipsychotic drugs, obesity, and diabetes. *J Clin Psychiatry* 65:267–272, 2004.

American Psychiatric Association. *Diagnostic and statistical manual of mental disorders* (4th ed., text rev.). Washington DC: Author, 2000. (Electronic version)

American Psychiatric Association. APA Task Force on electroconvulsive therapy. *The practice of electroconvulsive therapy: Recommendations for treatment, training, and privileging.* Washington, DC.: Author, 2001.

American Psychiatric Association. *Practice guidelines for the treatment of patients with schizophrenia (2nd ed.), 2004. Retrieved April 23, 2006, from www.psych.org/psych_pract/treatg/pg/prac_guide.cfm.*

American Psychiatric Association. *Assessing and treating suicidal behaviors: A quick reference guide. Retrieved February 6, 2006, from www.psych.org/psych_pract/treatg/quick_ref_guide/SuicidalBehaviorsQRG_04-15-05.pdf.*

Ames D, Ballard C, Cream J, Shah A, Suh GH, & McKeith I. For debate: Should novel antipsychotics ever be used to treat the behavioral and psychological symptoms of dementia (BPSD)? *International Psychogeriatrics* 17(1):3–29, 2005.

Andrezina R, Josiassen RC, Marcus RN, Oren DA, Manos G, Stock E, Carson WH, & Iwamoto T. Intramuscular aripiprazole for the treatment of acute agitation in patients with schizophrenia or schizoaffective disorder: A double-blind, placebo-controlled comparison with intramuscular haloperidol. *Psychopharmacology* 188:281–92, 2006.

Arieti S. *Interpretation of schizophrenia* (2nd ed). Lanham, MD: Jason Aronson, 1994.

Atkinson, JW. *Motives in fantasy, action, and society.* Princeton, NJ: Van Nostrand, 1958.

Bagby RM, Taylor GJ, Parker JDA, Dickens S. The development of the Toronto Structured Interview for Alexithymia: Item selection, factor structure, reliability, and concurrent validity. *Psychotherapy and Psychosomatics* 75:25–39, 2006.

Ballard C, Grace J, & Homes C. Neuroleptic sensitivity in dementia with Lewy bodies and Alzheimer's disease. *Lancet* 351(4):1032–3, 1998.

Bazan NG. *Lipid mediators in ischemic brain damage and experimental epilepsy.* Basel, Switzerland: Karger Press, 1990.

Beck AT, & Newman CF. Cognitive therapy. In BJ Sadock & VA Sadock (Eds.), *Kaplan & Sadock's comprehensive textbook of psychiatry* (Vol. II, 8th ed.). Philadelphia: Lippincott, Williams & Wilkins, 2005, pp. 2595–2610.

Birren, JE & Shaie KW (Eds). *Handbook of the psychology of aging* (5th ed.). New York: Academic Press, 2001.

Blank G, & Blank R. *Ego psychology II.* New York: Grune & Stratton, 1979.

Blazer DG. Hypochondriasis. In WB Abrams & Berkow (Eds.), *The Merck Manual of Geriatrics.* Rahway, NJ: Merck Sharp & Dohme Research Laboratories, 1990, pp. 1011–1018.

Borson S, Scanlan J, Brush M, Vitaliano P, & Dokmak A. The mini-cog: A cognitive "vital signs" measure for dementia screening in multilingual elderly. *Int J Ger Psychiatry* 15(11):1021–7, 2000.

Bourgeois MS, Camp C, Rose M, White B, Malone M, Carr J, & Rovine MA Comparison of training strategies to enhance use of external aids by persons with dementia. *J Commun Disord* 36:361–78, 2003.

Bowlby J. Attachment and loss: Loss, sadness, and depression (Vol. III). New York: Basic Books, 1980.

Bristol-Myers Squibb. Aripiprazole slide kit, 2002.

Brodaty H, Cullen B, Thompson C, Mitchell P, Parker G, Wilhelm K, Austin MP, Malhib, G. Age and gender in the phenomenology of depression. *Am J Ger Psychiatry* 13(7):589–96, 2005.

Brodaty H, & Finkel SI. *BPSD: Behavioral and psychological symptoms of dementia educational pack.* Skokie, IL: International Psychogeriatric Association (IPA), 2003. Also available at *www.ipa-online.org*.

Busch KA, & Fawcett J. A fine-grained study of inpatients who commit suicide. *Psychiatric Ann* 34:357–64, 2004.

Butler RN. The life review: An interpretation of reminiscence in the aged. *Psychiatry* 26:65–76, 1963.

Butler RN, & Lewis MI. *Aging and mental health: Positive psychosocial approaches.* St. Louis, MO: Mosby, 1977.

Cabeza R. Hemispheric asymmetry reduction in older adults: The HAROLD model. *Psychology & Aging* 17(3):1394–402, 2002.

Camp CJ. Montessori-based activities for persons with dementia (Vol. 1). Beachwood, OH: Menorah Park Center for the Aging, 1999.

Carolina Population Center. The Oakland Growth and Berkeley Guidance Studies of the Institute of Human Development at the University of California, Berkeley. Retrieved October 22, 2006, from *www.cpc.unc.edu/projects/life-course/oakland_berkeley*.

Carson S, McDonagh MS, Peterson K. A systematic review of the efficacy and safety of atypical antipsychotics in patients with psychological and behavioral symptoms of dementia. *Journal of the American Geriatrics Society* (JAGS) 54(2):354–361, 2006.

Cartwright, RD. Who needs their dreams?: The usefulness of dreams in psychoanalysis. *J Am Acad Psychoanalysis* 21:539–47, 1993.

Caspi A, Sugden K, Moffitt TE, Taylor A, Craig IW, Harnington H, et al. Influence of life stress on depression: Moderation by a polymorphism of the 5-HTT gene. *Science* 301(5631):386–9.

Centers for Disease Control. Chronic fatigue syndrome (CSF) basic facts. Retrieved October 7, 2006, from *www.cdc.gov/print.do?url=http://www.cdc.gov/cfs/cfs basicfacts.htm*.

Clark MR. Psychogenic disorders: A pragmatic approach for formulation and treatment. *Seminars in Neurology* 26(3):357–366, 2006.

Cheong JA. An evidence-based approach to the management of agitation in the geriatric patient. FOCUS 2(2):197–205, 2004.

Cochrane Collaboration Reviews. Retrieved December 1, 2005 from *www.cochrane.org/reviews*

Cohen GD. *The mature mind: The positive power of the aging brain.* New York: Basic Books, 2005.

Cohen G, & Taylor S. Reminiscence and ageing. *Ageing Society* 18:601–610, 1998.

Cohen GD. *The creative age: Awakening human potential in the second half of life.* New York: Harper-Collins, 2000.

Cohen-Mansfield J, Marx MS, & Rosenthal AS. A description of agitation in a nursing home. *J Gerontology* 44:M77–M87, 1989.

Cohen-Mansfield J. Non-pharmacologic interventions for inappropriate behaviors in dementia: A review, summary, and critique. *Am J Ger Psychiatry* 9:361–81, 2001.

Colarusso CA, & Nemiroff RA. Clinical implications of adult developmental theory. *Am J Psychiatry* 144:1263–70, 1987.

Coppen A, Abou-Saleh M, Milln P, Metcalf M, Harwood J, Bailey J. Dexamethasone suppression test in depression and other psychiatric illness. *Brit J Psychiatry* 142:498–504, 1983.

Coryell W, Nopoulos P, Drevets W, Wilson T, Andreasen NC. Subgenual prefrontal cortex volumes in major depressive disorder and schizophrenia: Diagnostic specificity and prognostic implications. *Am J of Psychiatry* 162:1706–1712, 2005.

Costa PT, Jr., & McCrae RR. *The NEO personality inventory manual.* Odessa, FL: Psychological Assessment Resources, 1985.

Cummings JL, & Back C. The cholinergic hypothesis of neuropsychiatric symptoms in Alzheimer's diseaes. *Am J Ger Psychiatry* 6:S64-S78, 1998.

Cummings JL, Mega M, Gray K, Rosenberg-Thompson L, Carusi DA, & Gornbein J. The neuropsychiatric inventory: Comprehensive assessment of psychopathology in dementia. *Neurology* 44:2308–14, 1994.

Dalvi A. Normal pressure hydrocephalus. *E-medicine.* Retrieved February 10, 2007 from *www.emedicine.com/neuro/topic277.htm.*

Day CR. Validation therapy: A review of the literature. *J Gerontological Nursing* 23:29–34, 1997.

Deutsch LH, Bylsma FW, Rover BW, Steele C, & Folstein MF. Psychosis and physical aggression in probable Alzheimer's disease. *Am J Psychiatry* 148(9):1159–63, 1991.

Duberstein PR, Conwell Y, Conner KR, Eberly S, & Caine ED. Suicide at 50 years of age and older: Perceived physical illness family discord and financial strain. *Psychol Med* 34:137–46, 2004.

Duke University Center for the Study of Aging and Human Development. Older adults: Resources and services. Retrieved October 22, 2006, from *www.geri.duke.edu/service/oars.htm.*

Egeland J, Lund A, Landro NI, Rund BR, Sundet K, Asbjornsen A, Mjellem N, Roness A, & Stordal KI. Cortisol level predicts executive and memory function in depression, symptom level predicts psychomotor speed. *Acta Psychiatr Scand* 112:434–41, 2005.

Elgh E, Astot AL, Fagerlund M, Eriksson S, Olsson T, & Nasman B. Cognitive dysfunction, hippocampal atrophy, and glucocorticoid feedback in Alzheimer's disease. *Biol Psychiatry* 59:155–61, 2006.

Ely EW, Inouye SK, Bernard GR, Gordon S, Francis J, May L, Truman B, Speroff T, Gautam S, Margoin R, Hart RP, & Dittus R. Delirium in mechanically ventilated patients: Validity and reliability of the confusion assessment method for the intensive care unit (CAM-ICU). *JAMA* 5:286(21), 2703–10, 2001.

Engel, GL. The need for a new medical model, *Science* 196:129–136, 1977.

Erdelyi MH. *Psychoanalysis: Freud's cognitive psychology.* New York: Freeman, 1985.

Erikson E. *Childhood and society.* New York: Norton, 1963.

Evans DL, Charney DS, Lewis L, Golden RN, Gorman JM, Krishnan KRRK,

Nemeroff CB, Bremner JD, Carney RM, et al. Mood disorders in the medically ill: Scientific review and recommendations. *Biol Psychiatry* 58:175–89, 2005.

Federal Drug Administration (FDA). Revisions to medication guide antidepressant medications, depression and other serious mental illnesses, and suicidal thoughts or actions. Retrieved September 14, 2007, from *www.fda.gov/cder/drug/antidepressants/antidepressants_MG_2007.pdf*

Feil N. The validation breakthrough. Cleveland, OH: Feil Productions, 2002.

Fields HL, & Martin JB. Pain: Pathophysiology and management. In BJ Sadock & VA Sadock (Eds.), *Comprehensive textbook of psychiatry* (7th ed.). Philadelphia: Lippincott, Williams & Wilkins, 2000.

Flaherty JH, & Morley JE. Anti-aging. *Clin Ger Med* 20(2), 2004.

Ford DE, & Kamerow DB. Epidemiologic study of sleep disturbances and psychiatric disorders. An opportunity for prevention? *JAMA* 262:1479–84, 1989.

Freud A. *The ego and the mechanisms of defense.* London: Hogarth Press and Institute of Psycho-Analysis, 1937.

Freud S. *Collected works of Sigmund Freud.* New York: Hogarth Press, 1986.

Francis J, Martin D, & Kapoor WN. A prospective study of delirium in hospitalized elderly. *JAMA* 263:1097–101, 1990.

Friedman JI, Harvey PD, Kemether E, Byne W, & Davis KL. Cognitive and functional changes with aging in schizophrenia. *Biol Psychiatry* 46:921–8, 1999.

Fries JF. Aging, natural death, and the compression of morbidity. *New Eng J Med* 303:130–135, 1980.

Fugh-Berman A. Alternative medicine. In DL Kasper, E Braunwald, A Fauci, S Hauser, & D Longo (Eds.), *Harrison's principles of internal medicine* (16th ed.). New York: McGraw-Hill, 2005, pp. 49–54.

The Gallup Organization. *Sleep in America: 1995 Gallup Poll conducted for the National Sleep Foundation.* Retrieved September 20, 2000, from *www.stanford.edu/~dement/95poll.html.*

Gendlin ET. *Focusing.* New York: Bantam Books, 1981.

Giese-Davis J, Dimiceli S, Sephton S, & Spiegel D. Emotional expression and diurnal cortisol slope in women with metastatic breast cancer in supportive–expressive group therapy: A preliminary study. *Biol Psycho* 73:190–8, 2006.

Greenblatt DJ, von Moltke, LL, Harmatz JS, Shader RI. Pharmacokinetics, pharmacodynamics, and drug disposition. In KL Davis, D Charney, JT Coyle, & C Nemeroff (Eds.), *Neuropsychopharmacology: The fifth generation of progress.* Philadelphia: Lippincott Williams & Wilkins, 2002, pp. 507–524.

Greenspan SI & Pollock GH (Eds.). *The course of life: Psychoanalytic contributions toward understanding personality development (Vol. III): Adulthood and the aging process.* DHHS Pub. (ADM) 81-1000, Washington, DC: Government Printing Office, 1980.

Grimley EJ, Malouf R, Huppert F, & van Niekerk J. Dehydroepiandrosterone (DHEA) supplementation for cognitive function in healthy elderly people. *Cochrane Database Syst Rev* (4):CD006221, Oct 18, 2006.

Grotjahn M. Analytic psychotherapy with the elderly. *Psychoanalytic Rev* 42(4):419–27, 1955.

Group for the Advancement of Psychiatry Committee on Aging. Medicare managed mental health care: A looming crisis. *Psychiatric Services* 56(7):795–8, 2005.

Gureje O, Simon GE, & Von Korff M. A cross-national study of the course of persistent pain in primary care. *Pain* 92(1–2):195–200, 2001.

Gurland BJ. Epidemiology of psychiatric disorders. In J Sadavoy, LF Jarvik, GT Grossberg, & BS Meyers (Eds.), *Comprehensive textbook of geriatric psychiatry* (3rd ed.). New York: Norton, 2004, pp. 3–37.

Hardy J. The genetics of neurodegenerative diseases. *J Neurochemistry* 97:1690–9, 2006.

Hardy J, & Selkoe DJ. The amyloid hypothesis of Alzheimer's disease: Progress and problems on the road to therapeutics. *Science* 297:353–6, 2002.

Harrison PJ, & Weinberger DR. Schizophrenia genes within cortical neural circuits. *Molecular Psychiatry* 10:5, 2005.

Harvey PD, Conference report: The seventh biennial Mt. Sinai Conference on cognition in schizophrenia. *Schizophrenia Bul* 31:895–7, 2005.

Harvey PD, & McClure MM. Pharmacologic approaches to the management of cognitive dysfunction in schizophrenia. *Drugs* 66:1466–73, 2006.

Harvey PD, Moriarty PJ, Bowie C, Friedman JI, Parrella M, White L, & Davis KL. Cortical and subcortical cognitive deficits in schizophrenia: Convergence of classifications based on language and memory skill areas. *J Clin Exp Neuropsychology* 24:55–66, 2002.

Hayflick L. The limited in vitro lifetime of human diploid cell strains. *Exp Cell Res* 37:614–36, 1965.

Hoehn, MM, & Yahr MD. Parkinsonism: Onset, progression, and mortality. *Neurology* 17: 427–442, 1967.

Hogarty GE, Flesher S, Ulrich R, Carter M, Greenwald D, Pogue-Geile M, Kechavan M, Cooley S, DiBarry LA, Garrett A, Parapally H, & Zoretich R. Cognitive enhancement therapy for schizophrenia: Effects of a 2-year randomized trial on cognition and behavior. *Arch Gen Psychiatry* 61:866–76, 2004.

Hollifield M, Tuttle L, Paine S, & Kellner R. Hypochondriasis and somatization related to personality and attitudes toward self. *Psychosomatics* 40:387–95, 1999.

Hollis J, Touyz S, Grayson D, & Forrester L. Antipsychotic medication dispensing and associated odds ratios of death in elderly veterans and war widows. *Australian New Zealand Psychiatry*, 40:981–6, 2006.

Horowitz, MJ, Bonanno GA, Holen A. Pathological grief: Diagnosis and explanation. *Psychosomatic Medicine* 55(3):260–273, 1993.

Insel TR. Beyond efficacy: The STAR*D Trial. *Am J Psychiatry* 163:5–7, 2006.

Institute of Medicine, Committee on Nursing Home Regulation. *Improving the quality of care in nursing homes.* Washington, DC: National Academy Press, 1986.

International Society for Interpersonal Psychotherapy. Introducing IPT into a mental health service. Retrieved October 7, 2006, from *www.interpersonalpsychotherapy.org/index.html.*

Jacobs GD, Pace-Schott EF, Stickgold R, & Otto MW. Cognitive behavior therapy and pharmacotherapy for insomnia. *Arch Intern Med* 164:1888–1896, 2004.

Jameson, JL. Principles of endocrinology. In E Braunwald, AS Fauci, DL Kasper, SL Hauser, DL Longo, & JL Jameson (Eds.), *Harrison's principles of internal medicine* (15th ed.). New York: McGraw Hill, 2001, pp. 2019–2029.

Jeste DV, Dunn LB, & Lindamer LA. Psychoses. In J Sadavoy, LF Jarvk, GT Grossberg, & BS Meyers (Eds.), *Comprehensive textbook of geriatric psychiatry* (3rd ed.). New York: Norton, 2004, pp. 655–685.

Jeste DV, Finkel SI. Psychosis of Alzheimer's disease and related dementias: Diagnostic criteria for a distinct syndrome. *Am J Ger Psychiatry* 8(1):29–34, 2000.

Jeste DV, Okamoto A, Napolitano J, Kane JM, & Martinez RA. Low incidence of persistent tardive dyskinesia in elderly patients with dementia treated with risperidone. *Am J Psychiatry* 157:1150–5, 2000.

Johnson CJ, & Johnson RH. Alzheimer's disease as a "trip back in time." *Am J Alzheimer's Disease* 15(2):87–93, 2000.

Jones PB, Barnes TRE, Davies L, Dunn G, Lloyd H, Hayhurst KP, Murray RM, Markwick A, & Lewis SW. Randomized controlled trial of the effect on quality of life of second- vs first-generation antipsychotic drugs in schizophrenia. *Arch Gen* Psychiatry 63:1079–87, 2006.

Jost BC, & Grossberg GT. The evolution of psychiatric symptoms in Alzheimer's disease: A natural history study. *J Am Ger Society* 45:891–2, 1996.

Kasper DL, Braunwald E, Fauci A, Hauser, S, Longo D (Eds). *Harrison's principles of internal medicine* (15th ed.). New York: McGraw-Hill, 2005.

Katz DA, & McHorney CA. Clinical correlates of insomnia in patients with chronic illness. *Arch Intern Med* 158:1099–1107, 1998.

Kay SR, Fiszbein A, & Opler LA. The positive and negative syndrome scale (PANSS) for schizophrenia. *Schizophrenia Bull* 13:261–76, 1987.

Kendler KS. Reflections on the relationship between psychiatric genetics and psychiatric nosology. *Am J Psychiatry* 163:1138–46, 2006.

Koenig HG. The role of religion/spirituality in the mental health of older adults. In J Sadavoy, LF Jarvik, GT Grossberg, & BS Meyers (Eds.), *Comprehensive textbook of geriatric psychiatry* (3rd ed.). New York: Norton, 2004, pp. 203–223.

Kwentus J. Sleep disorders in geriatric psychiatry. In J Sadavoy, LF Jarvik, GT Grossberg, & BS Meyers (Eds.), *Comprehensive textbook of geriatric psychiatry* (3rd ed.). New York: Norton, 2004, pp. 763–787.

Lavretsky H, & Nguyen LH. Diagnosis and treatment of neuropsychiatric symptoms in Alzheimer's disease. *Psychiatric Services* 57:617–19, 2006.

Lederberg MS, & Joshi N. End-of-life and palliative care. In BJ Sadock & VA Sadock (Eds.), *Kaplan & Sadock's comprehensive textbook of psychiatry* (8th ed., Vol II). Philadelphia: Lippincott, Williams & Wilkins, pp. 2336–2366, 2005.

Leszcz M. Group therapy. In J Sadavoy, LF Jarvik, GT Grossberg, & BS Meyers (Eds.), *Comprehensive textbook of geriatric psychiatry* (3rd ed.). New York: Norton, 2004, pp. 1023–1054.

Leventhal EA, & Burns EA. The biology of aging. In J Sadavoy, LF Jarvik, GT Grossberg, & BS Meyers (Eds.), *Comprehensive textbook of geriatric psychiatry* (3rd ed.). New York: Norton, 2004, pp. 105–130.

Levinson DJ, Darrow CN, & Klein EB. *The seasons of a man's life*. New York: Knopf, 1978.

Levkoff SE, Cleary P, Liptzin B, & Evans DA. Epidemiology of delirium: An overview of research issues and findings. *International Psychogeriatrics* 3:149–67, 1991.

Levkoff SE, Evans DA, Liptzin B, Cleary PD, Lipsitz LA, Wetle TT, Reilly CH, Pilgrim DM, Schor J, & Rowe J. Delirium. The occurrence and persistence of symptoms among elderly hospitalized patients. *Arch Int Med* 152:334–40, 1992.

Li G, Cherrier MM, Tsuang DW, Petrie EC, Colasurdo EA, Craft S,

Schellenberg GD, Peskind ER, Raskind MA, & Wilkinson CW. Salivary cortisol and memory function in human aging. *Neurobiology of Aging* 27(11):1705–1714, 2006.

Libon DJ, Xie SX, Moore P, Farmer J, Antani S, McCawley G, Cross K, & Grossman M. Patterns of neuropsychological impairment in frontotemporal dementia. *Neurology* 68:369–75, 2007.

Lieberman JA, Stroup TS, McEvoy JP, Swartz MS, Rosenheck RA, Perkins DO, Keefe RSE, Davis SM, Davis CE, Lebowitz BD, Severe J & Hsiao JK. Effectiveness of antipsychotic drugs in patients with chronic schizophrenia. *New England Journal of Medicine* 353:1209–23, 2005.

Linehan MM, Armstrong HE, Suarez A, Allmon D, & Heard HL. Cognitive-behavioral treatment of chronically parasuicidal borderline patients. *Arch Gen Psychiatry* 48:1060–4, 1991.

Lombardo ER, & Nezu AM. Medically unexplained symptoms. In A Freeman (Ed.), *Encyclopedia of cognitive behavior therapy.* New York: Springer, 2005, pp. 241–4.

Lukiw WJ, Cui JG, Marcheselli VL, Bodker M, Botkjaer A, Gotlinger, K, Serhan CH, & Bazan NG. A role for docosahexaenoic acid—derived neuroprotectin D1 in neural cell survival and Alzheimer disease. *J Clin Investigation* 115(10): 1–10, 2005.

Lynch TR, Morse JQ, Mendelson T, & Robins CJ. Dialectical behavior therapy for depressed older adults. *Am J Ger Psychiatry* 11:33–45, 2003.

Magri F, Cravello L, Barli L, Sarra S, Cinchetti W, Salmoiraghi F, Micale G, & Ferrari E. Stress and dementia: The role of the hypothalamic–pituitary–adrenal axis. *Aging Clin Exp Research* 18:167–70, 2006.

Manji HK, Quiroz JA, Payne JL, Singh J, Lopes BP, Viegas JS, & Zarate CA. The underlying neurobiology of bipolar disorder. *World Psychiatry* 2:136–46, 2003.

Marcantonio ER, Rudolph JL, Culley D, Crosby G, Alsop D, & Inouye SK. Serum biomarkers for delirium. *J Gerontology* 61A:1281–6, 2006.

Maslow AH. A theory of human motivation. *Psychol Rev* 50:370–96, 1943.

Mathuranath RM. Tau and tauopathis. *Neurology India* 55:11–16, 2007.

Mayou R, Kirmayer LJ, Simon G, Kroenke K, & Sharpe M. Somatoform disorders: Time for a new approach in DSM-V. *Am J Psychiatry* 162:847–55, 2005.

McClelland, DC. *Power: The inner experience.* New York: Halstead, 1975.

McClelland DC, Atkinson JW, Clark RA, & Lowell EL. *The achievement motive.* Princeton: Van Nostrand, 1953.

McCrae RR & Costa PT. *Personality in adulthood.* New York: Guilford Press, 1990.

McEwen BS, & Wingfield JC. The concept of allostasis in biology and biomedicine. *Hormones and Behavior* 43:2–15, 2003.

McFadden ER, Jr. Diseases of the respiratory system. In E Braunwald, A Fauci, DL Kasper, SL Hauser, DL Longo, JL Mameson (Eds). *Harrison's principles of internal medicine* (15th ed.). New York: McGraw-Hill, 2001, pp. 1456–1463.

McKhann G, Drachman D, Folstein M, Katzman R, Price D, & Stadlan EM. Clinical diagnosis of Alzheimer's disease: Report of the NINCDS-ADRDA Work Group under the auspices of Department of Health and Human Services Task Force on Alzheimer's Disease. *Neurology* 34:939–44, 1984.

McShane R. What are the syndromes of behavioral and psychological symptoms of dementia? *International Psychogeriatrics* 12(1): 147–53, 2000.

Medical Care Corporation. Differential diagnostic workup of Alzheimer's disease and related disorders. Retrieved December 3, 2006, from *www.mccare.com/diagnostic_criteria.jsp*.

Meehan K, Zhang F, David S, Tohen M, Janicak P, Small J, Koch K, Rizk R, Walker D, Tran P, & Breier A. A double-blind, randomized comparison of the efficacy and safety of intramuscular injections of olanzapine, lorazepam, or placebo in treating acutely agitated patients diagnosed with bipolar mania. *J Clin Psychopharmacology* 21:389–97, 2001.

Mega MS, Cummings JL, Fiorello T, & Gornbein J. The spectrum of behavioral changes in Alzheimer's disease. *Neurology* 46:130–135.

Mendoza J. *Comparing early dementia syndromes.* Handout from the New Orleans VA Medical Center, August 7, 2005.

Meyers JK, Weissman MM, Tischler GL, Holzer CE III, Leaf PJ, Orvaschel H, Anthony JC, Boyd JH, Burke JD Jr, Kramer M, & Stoltzman R. Six-month prevalence of psychiatric disorders in three communities 1980–1982. *Arch Gen Psychiatry* 41(10):959–67, 1984.

Moran M. Trauma, cancer patients have much in common. *Psychiatric News* 39(14):26, 2004. Retrieved September 10, 2006, from *pn.psychiatryonline.org/cgi/content/full/39/14/26*.

Morrison G, O'Carroll R, & McCreadie R. Long-term course of cognitive impairment in schizophrenia. *British J of Psychiatry*, 189:556–57, 2006.

Munetz MR, & Benjamin S. How to examine patients using the Abnormal Involuntary Movement Scale. *Hospital and Community Psychiatry* 39(11):1172–7, 1988.

Munoz RF, & Miranda J. *Group therapy manual for cognitive behavioral treatment of depression.* Santa Monica, CA: RAND, 2000.

NAMI NH. Mental health, mental illness, healthy aging: A New Hampshire guidebook for older adults and caregivers. Concord, NH: NAMI, December, 2001.

National Cancer Institute normal adjustment and the adjustment disorders. Retrieved September 10, 2006, from *www.nci.nih.gov/cancertopics/pdq/supportivecare/adjustment/healthprofessional*.

National Heart, Lung & Blood Institute. Body mass index table. Retrieved September 8, 2007, from *www.nhibi.nih.gov/guidelines/obesity/bmi_tbl.htm*

National Institute on Aging. Baltimore Longitudinal Study on Aging (BLSA). Retrieved March 5, 2007, from *www.grc.nia.nih.gov/branches/blsa/blsanew.htm*.

National Institute of Mental Health. Older adults: Depression and suicide facts. Retrieved February 20, 2007, from *www.nimh.nih.gov/publicat/elderlydepsuicide.cfm*.

National Institute of Neurological Disorders and Stroke (NINDS). Dementia with lewy bodies information page. Retrieved February 20, 2007, from *www.ninds.nih.gov/disorders/dementiawithlewybodies/dementiawithlewybodies.htm*.

National Institute of Neurological Disorders and Stroke (NINDS). Frontotemporal dementia information page. Retrieved February 20, 2007, from *www.ninds.nih.gov/disorders/picks/picks.htm*.

National Institute of Neurological Disorders and Stroke (NINDS). Restless legs syndrome fact sheet. Retrieved February 20, 2007, *from www.ninds.nih.gov/disorders/restless_legs/detail_restless_legs.htm*

National Institute of Neurological Disorders and Stroke (NINDS). Sleep apnea Information Page. Retrieved February 22, 2007, from *www.ninds.nih.gov/disorders/sleep_apnea/sleep_apnea.htm*.

National Parkinson Association. The Unified Parkinson Disease Rating Scale. Retrieved February 1, 2007, from *www.parkinson.org/site/pp.asp?c= 9dJFJLPwB&b=100016*.

Nemiroff RA, & Colarusso CA. *The race against time: Psychotherapy and psychoanalysis in the second half of life*. New York: Plenum Press, 1985.

Neugarten BL. Time, age, and the life cycle. Am J *Psychiatry* 136(7):887–94, 1979.

O'Brien JT, Lloyd A, McKeith I, Gholkar A, & Ferrier N. A longitudinal study of hippocampal volume, cortisol levels, and cognition in older depressed subjects. *Am J Psychiatry* 161:2081–90, 2004.

Online Mendelian Inheritance in Man (OMIM). Frontotemporal dementia. Retrieved February 20, 2007, from *www.ncbi.nlm.nih.gov/entrez/dispomin.cgi?id=600274*.

Pandharipande P, Shintani A, Peterson J, Pun BT, Wilkinson GR, Dittus RS, Bernard GR, & Ely EW. Lorazepam is an independent risk factor for transitioning to delirium in intensive care patients. *Anesthesiology* 104(1):21–26, 2006.

Patterson CH. Understanding psychotherapy. *Fifty years of client centered theory and practice*. Ross-on-Wye, UK: PCCS Books, 2000.

Polymeropoulos, MH, Lavedan C, Leroy E, Ide SE, Dehejia A, Dutra A, et. al. Mutation in the α-synclein gene identified in families with Parkinson's disease. *Science* 276(5321):2045–47, 1997.

PROSPECT (Prevention of Suicide in Primary Care Collaborative Trial). Retrieved January 15, 2006, from *www.hhs.gov/asl/testify/t000208b.html*

Reisberg B. Functional assessment staging (FAST). *Psychopharm Bulletin* 24(4): 653–59, 1984.

Reite M, Ruddy J, & Nagel K. *Concise guide to evaluation and management of sleep disorders* (3rd ed.). Washington, DC: American Psychiatric Press, 2002.

Reynolds J, & Mintzer J. Alzheimer disease update: New targets, new options. *Drug Benefit Trends* 17:83–88, 91–95, 2005.

Richelson E. Receptor pharmacology of neuroleptics: Relation to clinical effects. *J Clin Psychiatry* 60(10):5–14, 1999.

Richelson E. Pharmacology of antidepressants. *Mayo Clinic Proceedings* 76:511–27, 2001.

Richelson E. Interactions of antidepressants with neurotranmitter transporters and receptors and their clinical relevance. *J Clin Psychiatry* 64(13):5–12, 2003.

Riegel KF. The dialectics of human development. *American Psychologist* 31:689–700, 1976.

Rogaeva E, Meng Y, Lee JH, Gu Y, Kawarai T, Zou F, Katayama T, Baldwin CT, Cheng R, Hasegawa H, Chen F, Shibata N, et al. The neuronal sortilin-related receptor SORL1 is genetically associated with Alzheimer's disease. *Nature Genetics* 39:168–177, 2007.

Roman GC, Tatemichi TK, Erkinjuntti T, Cummings JL, et al. Vascular dementia: Diagnostic criteria for research studies. Report of the NINDS-AIREN International Workshop 43:250–60, 1993.

Rosen WG, Mohs RC, & Davis KL. A new rating scale for Alzheimer's disease (ADAS). *Am J Psychiatry* 141:1356–64, 1984.

Royal D. Personal communication. (2007).

Rubert MP, Lowenstein DA, & Eisdorfer C. Normal aging: Changes in cognitive abilities. In J Sadavoy, LF Jarvik, GT Grossberg, & BS Meyers (Eds.), *Comprehensive textbook of geriatric psychiatry* (3rd ed.). New York: Norton, 2004, pp. 131–46.

Rubin JJ. Psychosomatic pain: New insights and management strategies. *Southern Medical Journal* 98(11): 1099–110, 2005.

Rudorfer M, Henry ME, & Sackeim HA. Electroconvulsive therapy. In A Tasman, JA Lieberman, & J Fletcher (Eds.), *Psychiatry*. New York: Saunders, 1997.

Sadavoy J, & Lazarus LW. Individual psychotherapy. In J Sadavoy, LF Jarvik, GT Grossberg, & BS Meyers (Eds.), *Comprehensive textbook of geriatric psychiatry* (3rd ed.). New York: Norton, 2004, pp. 993–1022.

Sadock BJ & VA (Eds). *Comprehensive textbook of psychiatry* (8th ed.). Baltimore: Lippincott Williams & Wilkins, 2004.

Sááez-Fonseca JA, Lee L, Walker Z. Long-term outcome of depressive pseudodementia in the elderly. *J of Aff Disorders* 101(1–3):129–9, 2007.

Sakauye KM, & Camp CJ. Introducing psychiatric care into nursing homes. *The Gerontologist* 32:849–52, 1992.

Saper CB, Chou TC, & Scammell TE. The sleep switch: Hypothalamic control of sleep and wakefulness. *Trends in Neurosciences (Review)* 24:726–31, 2001.

Schneider LS, Dagerman KS, & Insel P. Risk of death with atypical antipsychotic drug treatment for dementia: Meta-analysis of randomized placebo-controlled trials. *JAMA* 294:1934–43, 2005.

Schneider LS, Tariot PN, Dagerman KS, Davis SM, Hsiao JK, Ismail S, Lebowitz BD, Lyketsos CG, Ryan JM, Stroup TS, Sultzer DL, Weintraub D, & Lieberman JA. Effectiveness of atypical antipsychotic drugs in patients with Alzheimer's disease. *New Eng J Med* 355:1525–38, 2006.

Seaton G. *The crisis in nursing homes.* Wexford, Ireland: Adverbage Ltd., 2002.

Seligman MEP. *Helplessness: On depression, development, and death.* San Francisco: Freeman, 1975.

Seligman MEP. *Learned optimism.* New York: Simon & Schuster, 1998.

Selye H. *The stress of life.* New York: McGraw Hill, 1956/1978.

Sheehy G. *Passages: Predictable crises of adult life.* New York: Bantam Books, 1984.

Small JA, & Gutman G. Recommended and reported use of communication strategies in Alzheimer caregiving. *Alzheimer Disease and Associated Disorders* 16(4):270–8, 2002.

Soares JC, & Mann J. The functional neuroanatomy of mood disorders. *J Psychiatric Res* 31:393–432, 1997.

Soreq H. Simple blood test will accurately diagnose anxiety. Retrieved October 11, 2005, from *www.isracast.com*

Spitzer RL, Kroenke K, & Williams JB. Validation and utility of a self-report version of PRIME-MD: The PHQ primary care study. *JAMA* 282:1737–44, 1999.

Stahis SM. Delirium. *Essential psychopharmacology: Neuroscientific basis and practical applications* (2nd ed.). New York: Cambridge University Press, 2000.

Steffens DC, McQuoid DR, & Krishnan KR. The Duke somatic treatment algorithm for geriatric depression (STAGED) approach. *Psychopharmacology Bull* 36(2):58–68, 2002.

Steffens DC, Skoog I, Norton MC, Hart AD, Tschanz JT, Plassman BL, Wyse BW, Welsh-Bohmer A, & Breitner JCS. Prevalence of depression and its treatment in an elderly population: The Cache County Study. *Arch Gen Psychiatry* 57:601–07, 2000.

Stewart J. Allostatic load and allostasis. Retrieved August 12, 2006, from *www.macses.ucsf.edu/Research/Allostatic/notebook/allostatic.html*.

Streim JE, & Katz IR. Psychiatric aspects of long-term care. In J Sadavoy, LF Jarvik, GT Grossberg, & BS Meyers (Eds.), *Comprehensive textbook of geriatric psychiatry* (3rd ed.). New York: Norton, 2004, pp. 1071–102.

Suh GH, Greenspan AJ, & Choi SK. Comparative efficacy of risperidone versus haloperidol on behavioral and psychological symptoms of dementia. *Int J Ger Psychiatry* 21:654–60, 2006.

Tadafumi K. Mitochondrial dysfunction as the molecular basis of bipolar disorder: Therapeutic implications. *CNS Drugs* 21(1):1–11, 2007.

Takada Y, Yonezawa A, Kume T, Katsuki H, Kaneko S, Sugimoto H, & Akaike A. Nicotinic acetylcholine receptor-mediated neuroprotection by donepezil against glutamate neurotoxicity in rat cortical neurons. *J Pharm Exp Therapeutics*, 306:772–7, 2003.

Tariot PN, Farlow MR, Grossbert GT, Graham SM, McDonald S, & Gergel I. Memantine treatment in patients with moderate to severe Alzheimer disease already receiving donepezil: A randomized controlled trial. *JAMA* 291:317–24, 2004.

Taylor GJ, Bagby RM, & Parker JDA. *Disorders of affect regulation: Alexithymia in medical and psychiatric illness.* New York: Cambridge University Press, 1999.

Taylor P. Anticholinesterase agents. In JE Hardman, LE Limbird, & AG Gilman (Eds), *Goodman & Gilman's the pharmacological basis of therapeutics* (10th ed.). New York: McGraw-Hill, pp. 175–91, 2001.

Teeter RB, Garetz FK, Miller WR, & Hieland WF. Psychiatric disturbances of aged patients in skilled nursing homes. *Am J Psychiatry* 133:1430–4, 1976.

Texas Department of State Health Services. Texas Medication Algorithm Project (TMAP). Retrieved April 13, 2006, from *www.dshs.state.tx.us/mhprograms/disclaimer.shtm*.

Tran-Johsnson TK, Sack DA, Marcus RN, Auby P, McQuade RD, & Oren DA. Efficacy and safety of intramuscular aripiprazole in patients with acute agitation: A randomized, double-blind, placebo-controlled trial. *J Clin Psychiatry* 68:111–9, 2007.

Travedi MH, AJ Rush, SR Wisniewski, AA Nierenberg, D Warden, L Ritz, N Grayson, et. al. Evaluation of outcomes with citalopram for depression using measurement-based care in STAR*D: Implications for clinical practice. *Am J Psychiatry* 163:28–40, 2006.

Trepacz PT, Teague GB, & Lipowski ZJ. Delirium and other organic mental disorders in a general hospital. *General Hospital Psychiatry* 7:101–6, 1985.

Turvey CL, Conwell Y, Jones MP, Phillips C, Simonsick E, Pearson JL, & Wallace R. Risk factors for late-life suicide: A prospective, community-based study. *Am J Ger Psychiatry* 10(4):398–406, 2002.

U.S. Census Bureau (2000). Census 2000 gateway. Retrieved August 20, 2003, from www.census.gov/main/www.cen2000.html.

U.S. Department of Health and Human Services. *Mental health: Culture, race, and ethnicity — A supplement to mental health: A report of the Surgeon General.* Rockville, MD: U.S. Department of Health and Human Services, Substance Abuse and Mental Health Services Administration, Center for Mental Health Services, 2001.

U.S. Food and Drug Administration. Revisions to product labeling: Suicidality and antidepressant drugs. Retrieved February 20, 2007, from *www.fda.gov/cder/drug/antidepressants/antidepressants_label_change_2007.pdf*.

U.S. Food and Drug Administration. FDA talk paper T05-19: FDA approves Requip for restless legs syndrome. Retrieved December 20, 2006, from *www.fda.gov/bbs/topics/ANSWERS/2005/ANS01356.html.*

Vaillant GE. Aging well: *Surprising guideposts to a happier life from the landmark Harvard study of adult development.* New York: Little, Brown, 2003.

Vaillant GE. *Ego mechanisms of defense: A guide for clinicians and researchers.* Washington DC: American Psychiatric Press, Inc., 1992.

Vaillant GE. *Empirical studies of ego mechanisms of defense.* Washington DC: American Psychiatric Press, Inc., 1986.

Vaillant GE, & Mukamal K. Successful aging. *Am J Psychiatry* 158(6):839–47, 2001.

VanGerpen MW, Johnson JE, & Winstead DK. Mania in the geriatric patient population: A review of the literature. *Am J Ger Psychiatry* 7(3):188–202, 1999.

Vernon SD & Reeves WC. The challenge of integrating disparate high-content data: Epidemiological, clinical, and laboratory data collected during an in-hospital study of chronic fatigue syndrome. *Psychogenomics* 7(3):345–54, 2006.

Watson S, Thompson JM, Ritchie JC, Nicol FI, & Young AH. Neuropsychological impairment in bipolar disorder: The relationship with glucocorticoid receptor function. *Bipolar Disorder* 8:85–90, 2006.

Webster J, & Grossberg GT. Late-life onset of psychotic symptoms. *Am J Ger Psychiatry* 6(3):196–202, 1998.

Weisler RH, Barbee JG IV, & Townsend MH. Mental health and recovery in the Gulf Coast After Hurricanes Katrina and Rita. *JAMA* 296:585–8, 2006.

Wells CE. Pseudodementia. *Am J Psychiatry* 136:894–900, 1979.

Wells KB, Katon W, Robers B, & Camp P. Use of minor tranquilizers and antidepressant medications by depressed outpatients: Results from the medical outcomes study. *Am J Psychiatry* 151:697–700, 1994.

Werner P, Cohen-Mansfield J, Braun J, & Marx MS. Physical restraint and agitation in nursing home residents. *J Am Ger Soc* 37:1122–6, 1989.

Whistler T, Taylor R, Craddock RC, Broderick G, Klimas N, & Unger ER. Gene expression correlates of unexplained fatigue. *Psychogenomics* 7(3):395–405, 2006.

Witkowski JA. The postgenomic era and complex disease. *Pharmacogenomics* 7(3):341–343, 2006.

Woods B, Spector A, Jones C, Orrell M, Davies S. Reminiscence therapy for dementia. The Cochrane Database of Systematic Reviews 2005, Issue 2. Art. No.: CD001120.pub2. DOI: 10.1002/14651858.CD001120.pub2. *http://www.update-software.com/Abstracts/AB001120.htm* (accessed 2/23/06).

Worden JW. *Grief counseling and grief therapy: A handbook for the mental health practitioner.* New York: Springer, 1982.

Yousef G, Ryan WJ, Lambert T, Pitt B, & Kellett J. A preliminary report: A new scale to identify pseudodementia syndrome. *Int J Ger Psychiatry* 13:389–99, 1998.

Zola-Morgan S, & Squire LR. Neuroanatomy of memory. *Annual Review of Neuroscience* 16:547–563, 1993.

INDEX